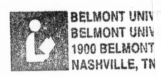

Manual
of Stroke
Rehabilitation

Physical Medicine and Rehabilitation Clinical Practice Manuals

Daxid X. Cifu, M.D., *Series Editor*

Manual
of Stroke
Rehabilitation

Karl J. Sandin, MD

Medical Director for Clinical Services,
The Rehabilitation Institute at Santa Barbara

Kristin D. Mason, MD

Staff Physiatrist and Team Leader,
Comprehensive Rehabilitation Program,
The Rehabilitation Institute at Santa Barbara

Butterworth–Heinemann

Boston • Oxford • Melbourne • Singapore • Toronto •
Munich • New Dehli • Tokyo

Every effort has been made to ensure that the drug dosage schedules within this text are accurate and conform to standards accepted at time of publication. However, as treatment recommendations vary in the light of continuing research and clinical experience, the reader is advised to verify drug dosage schedules herein with information found on product information sheets. This is especially true in cases of new or infrequently used drugs.

∞ Recognizing the importance of preserving what has been written, Butterworth–Heinemann prints its books on acid-free paper whenever possible.

Library of Congress Cataloging-in-Publication Data
Sandin, Karl J.
    Manual of stroke rehabilitation / Karl J. Sandin, Kristin D. Mason.
        p.   cm. — (Physical medicine and rehabilitation clinical practice manuals)
    Includes bibliographical references and index.
    ISBN 0-7506-9489-0   (alk. paper)
        1. Cerebrovascular disease—Patients—Rehabilitation—Handbooks, manuals, etc.   I. Mason, Kristin D.   II. Title.   III. Series.
        [DNLM: 1. Cerebrovascular Disorders—rehabilitation.   WL 355
    S217m 1996]
RC388.5.S187   1996
616.8'1--dc20
DNLM/DLC   95-44678
for Library of Congress   CIP

British Library Cataloguing-in-Publication Data
A catalogue record for this book is available from the British Library.

The publisher offers discounts on bulk orders of this book.
For information, please write:

Manager of Special Sales
Butterworth–Heinemann
313 Washington Street
Newton, MA 02158–1626

10 9 8 7 6 5 4 3 2 1

Printed in the United States of America

Contents

Contributing Authors

Sue Ellen Adams, OTR
Director of Occupational Therapy, The Rehabilitation Institute
at Santa Barbara

Joyce Gauvain, MA, CCC-SP
Manager, Speech/Language Pathology Department, The
Rehabilitation Institute at Santa Barbara

Kristin D. Mason, MD
Staff Physiatrist and Team Leader, Comprehensive Rehabilitation
Program, The Rehabilitation Institute at Santa Barbara

Kathryn H. Richmond, MS, RTR, CTRS
Director of Therapeutic Recreation, The Rehabilitation Institute
at Santa Barbara

Karl J. Sandin, MD
Medical Director for Clinical Services, The Rehabilitation
Institute at Santa Barbara

Ann E. Veazey, MS, PT
Director of Physical Therapy, The Rehabilitation Institute
at Santa Barbara

Preface

Stroke is the third leading cause of death and disability in the United States. Few lives have not in some way been touched by this disabling disease. Although modern medicine has eradicated or greatly curtailed many diseases, the incidence of stroke continues without significant change. Many stroke patients require specialized rehabilitation to return to as productive and meaningful lives as possible.

Overall we hope the information here will equip the reader with important knowledge that can be used to manage systems of stroke rehabilitation care, which, like health care in general, are in flux. Although multiauthored texts from multiple centers have their place, this book describes the care model at The Rehabilitation Institute at Santa Barbara, a not-for-profit, regional, freestanding hospital that provides acute and subacute rehabilitation, transitional living, home health care, and outpatient services. By focusing on a solitary rehabilitation system of stroke care, the reader is given a cogent whole, without the duplication and omission often seen in multicenter descriptions. We wrote these chapters bearing in mind our long experience with managed care in California. In some locations, managed-care organizations have not adequately utilized stroke rehabilitation; we believe that we have developed effective linkages with managed-care providers that ensure our continuing viability and patients' access to rehabilitation. It is our hope that these experiences will empower other rehabilitation providers to seek similar mutually beneficial alliances and affiliations with managed care organizations.

The *Manual of Stroke Rehabilitation* is designed to be comprehensive without being encyclopedic. The case studies are intended to amplify treatment discussions. The therapist responses give a different slant on physician-authored materials. This book is intended for the health-care professional who possesses some knowledge of rehabilitation and stroke. Particularly we hope that medical students; graduate medical trainees in rehabilitation, neurology, internal medicine, family practice, and other specialties; allied health students, practitioners, and managers; rehabilitation and nursing home administrators; managed-care administrators; and payers will find the information here interesting and useful in their work with stroke survivors.

KJS
KDM

Acknowledgments

We appreciate the confidence shown in us by David Cifu, M.D., series editor, who initially asked me, KJS, to write this textbook. We thank the editorial staff at Butterworth–Heinemann, especially Susan Pioli and Michelle St. Jean-Richards, for professionally assisting us with manuscript preparation.

Special thanks to the Rehabilitation Medical Group of the Central Coast. Our physician partners granted us flexibility so that we might concentrate on preparation of the manuscript. The wonderful administrative staff including Marisa Becerra, Elizabeth Muraoka, Lorraine Miner, Rae Jean Leu, Jill Meredith, and the now-retired Jan Cronk, faithfully typed, edited, fielded calls, and retrieved information.

We also appreciate the staff of The Rehabilitation Institute at Santa Barbara, including the four therapist contributors to this effort. Melinda Staveley, Vice President for Clinical Services at The Rehabilitation Institute at Santa Barbara provided expert review of Chapter 11, bringing her experience as the former Associate Director of the Commission on Accreditation of Rehabilitation Facilities to bear on this concluding segment. We are fortunate to work with such a fine, dedicated group, people who are clearly called to the special work of rehabilitation. The Institute's patients are ably cared for by these outstanding individuals. We realize that we are privileged to serve those confronting disabling illnesses and impairments and, in turn, are honored by their hard work and determination in meeting adversity. This book is dedicated to these stroke survivors, their families, and caregivers.

KJS
KDM

On a personal note, I am indebted to so many professors from my years at Northwestern University Medical School and Baylor College of Medicine. They equipped me with tools for scientific inquiry and honed my skills in diagnosis and leadership. Knowing I cannot possibly mention all of them, I particularly want to thank Henry Betts, M.D., Elliot Roth, M.D., Martin Grabois, M.D., Susan J. (Jan) Garrison, M.D., Barry Smith, M.D., and William Donovan, M.D.

KJS

Stroke

Furious, frantic, downed as a flash-flooded
   oak, her left hand didn't wither, but dropped
     in a second all its green leaves,
her left leg shriveled to a seeming-useless wire,
   worthless as a severed root—

hope dried like cracked vines in an old, old
   Italian garden, crookedly weaving between toppled
     statues of children, young women, staring
at dirt, not daring to wish for rain, wind
   or the next day, or any day—

but pith-deep in this woman, iron, water
   mixed to explode, pushed sap back through
     kinked, flaking canals of brain,
     refueled stuttering cell fires—

and after weeks of sun and dark,
   low-banked steady fury,
   her hand undulates in the light,
she steps again with a walker down the street.

Ron Linder, MD©
San Francisco, California

(From *The Western Journal of Medicine*, 159(5):593, 1993. Used
with permission from the publisher and the author.)

1

Epidemiology and Pathophysiology

Stroke is a leading cause of death and disability for men and women of all ages, classes, and ethnic origins. In the United States, 500,000 new strokes occur each year, causing 150,000 deaths (the third leading cause of death overall, the second leading cause of death for women) and significant residual disability for many survivors[1,2] (Figure 1.1). Improvements in medical care have resulted in a steady decline in the stroke death rate over the past twenty years although the actual number of strokes appears to be increasing. Three million stroke survivors are alive today.

The word "stroke" applies to both *ischemic* (caused by decreased blood flow leading to infarction of tissue and cell injury and death) and *hemorrhagic* (cellular injury secondary to extravasation of blood into brain tissue) cerebrovascular disease, with either permanent or transient symptoms (Figure 1.2). Ischemic strokes are divided by pathophysiologic mechanism into thrombotic and embolic types. *Thrombotic* strokes, which are more common, develop in narrowed cerebral vessels and *embolic* strokes are caused by migration of material to central nervous system blood vessels from some distant source causing vascular occlusion and ischemia of brain tissue.

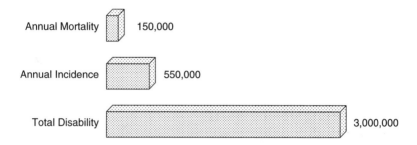

Annual Mortality   150,000

Annual Incidence   550,000

Total Disability   3,000,000

FIGURE 1.1   *Mortality, incidence, and disability from stroke, 1988.*

(Adapted from Stroke Clin Update III:1, 1992. Used with permission of the National Stroke Association, Englewood, CO.)

Thrombotic strokes are commonly associated with risk factors, such as hypertension, diabetes mellitus, and lipid disturbances, and tend to have a slower, stuttering, and more indolent onset. Embolic strokes are commonly associated with cardiac disease, such as atrial fibrillation and other dysrhythmias, valvular disease, or myocardial infarction, and tend to occur more suddenly. Because one cannot always determine the origin of an ischemic stroke, the term *thromboembolic* stroke is often preferred to describe the continuum seen in cerebral infarction.

Intracranial *hemorrhage* often presents more dramatically than ischemic stroke with headache and sudden neurologic deficits and can also cause vomiting, elevated blood pressure, and a decreased level of consciousness. In contrast with thromboembolic stroke, fluctuation in symptoms is rarely seen in hemorrhagic stroke. Patients with hemorrhage are often critically ill. Those who survive the initial injury often have more neurologic and functional recovery because the extravasated blood may only irritate neurons rather than causing cell death as with thromboembolic stroke. Hemorrhage may be into the brain tissue (*intraparenchymal* hemorrhage) or into the spaces lining the brain (*subarachnoid* hemorrhage). Intraparenchymal hemorrhage is generally caused by rupture of small arterioles in the basal ganglia, thalamus, cerebellum, or brain stem; is often associated with hypertension; and usually presents with sudden onset hemiparesis. Subarachnoid hemorrhage is usually caused by aneurysmal rupture and presents with decreased level of consciousness, headache, and meningismus (stiff neck), generally without lateralizing weakness.

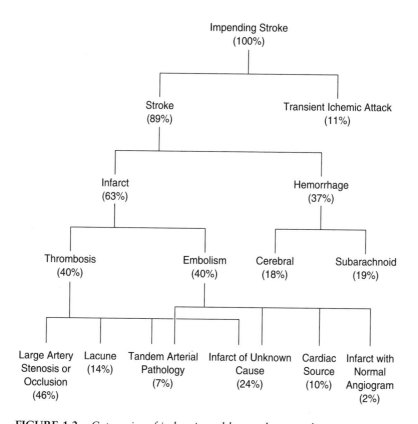

FIGURE 1.2   *Categories of ischemic and hemorrhage stroke.*

(Adapted from Grotta J. Acute stroke management. Stroke Clin Update III:18, 1993. Used with permission of the National Stroke Association, Englewood, CO.)

Ten percent of patients who present with focal neurologic signs compatible with stroke are found to sustain short-lived injury such as transient ischemic attacks (TIA) and reversible ischemic neurologic deficits (RIND). Although these patients often do not require hospitalization, they do need thorough evaluation; lifestyle modification; and institution of appropriate antiplatelet, cardiac, and other medications.

Specific arteries feed discrete areas of the brain. Interruption in cerebral circulation because of stroke results in classic stroke syndromes, which are described in Table 1.1. Table 1.2 lists lacunar syndromes.

TABLE 1.1   Stroke Syndromes

Artery	Presentation	Comments
Anterior Circulation		
Internal carotid	Face and arm > leg hemiparesis Hemisensory loss Homonymous hemianopsia Gaze preference to side of lesion Horner's syndrome on opposite side of lesion	Dominant hemisphere—aphasia Nondominant hemisphere—neglect
Middle cerebral	Face and arm > leg hemiparesis Hemispheric loss Gage preference	Most frequently involved Broca's (expressive) aphasia in upper-division infarction Wernick's (receptive) aphasia in lower-division infarction
Anterior cerebral	Leg > face and arm hemiparesis Hemispheric loss	
Venticulo-striate	Dense hemiparesis Dense hemisphere loss	Deep penetrating branches of MCA Hemorrhagic or lacunar
Posterior Circulation		
Posterior cerebral	Bilateral involvement—memory loss, vertigo, cortical blindness, prospagnosia Unilateral—homonynous, hemianopsia with macular sparing	
Basilar artery	Involves mid-brain, pons, and medulla Complete injury—locked-in syndrome with quadriplegia, bulbar plegia	Multiple syndromes

Posterior inferior cerebellar	Lateral medullary syndrome of Wallenberg:
	  ipsilateral Horner's
	  contralateral loss of pain and temperature over body
	  hoarseness
	  dysphagia
	  lower cranial nerve palsies
		Wallenberg syndrome also seen in other lesions

Anteroinferior cerebellar	Wallenberg and ipsilateral tinnitus and deafness	
Superior cerebellar artery	Pontomesencephalic injury	Varied brainstem presentation

TABLE 1.2 Lacunar Syndromes

Other Syndromes

Lacunar

Pure motor hemiparesis	Involves face, arm, and leg without sensory, visual or language loss
Pure hemisensory loss	Numbness of face, arm and leg without weakness, visual or language loss
Clumsy hand/dysarthria	Dysarthria, facial weakness, ipsilateral clumsiness of hand
Ataxia/hemiparesis	Cerebellar ataxia of arm and leg on one side, weakness of leg distally
Etat lacunaire	Because of multiple lacunes
Pseudobulbar palsy	Because of multiple strokes resulting in: bilateral corticospinal reflex signs spastic dysarthria dysphagia emotionalism

May lead to:
*Multi-infarct
dementia*

Modifiable risk factors for stroke include hypertension, diabetes mellitus, cardiac dysrhythmia (especially atrial fibrillation[2]), smoking,[3] obesity, hypercholesterolemia, and autoimmune disease.[4] Additionally, men, blacks, and those with a family history of cerebrovascular disease are more prone to stroke. Mitral annular calcification in the elderly and mitral prolapse in the young have been recognized as risk factors for stroke.[5,6] Trauma and medical interventions for other disorders, such as thrombolysis for myocardial infarction, have been linked to stroke.[7]

Stroke remains a significant threat to public health particularly for people of color and for people living in the U.S. "stroke belt," which runs across the Midwest and Southeast.[8] Probable factors for increased incidence in those groups include diets high in salt and fat, greater tobacco use among men, and higher rates of obesity and hypertension for black women. Yet blacks have a higher estimated incidence of stroke than whites even after adjustment for age, hypertension, and diabetes mellitus.[9] Young and middle-aged blacks have a substantially higher risk for subarachnoid or intracerebral hemorrhage than whites of similar age. These types of stroke are important causes of excess mortality among young and middle-aged blacks.[10] Klatsky et al. support this conclusion and note that blacks were at higher risk for hospitalization than whites for hemorrhagic cerebrovascular disease, cerebral thrombosis, and nonspecific cerebrovascular disease, but at lower hospitalization risk for extracranial occlusive disease.[11] Research continues on these poorly understood differences in stroke risk for whites and people of color.

Recent research has focused on two discrete groups that experience strokes. *Users of cocaine and other drugs* are at increased risk for stroke as well as seizures and behavioral abnormalities.[12] Cocaine-associated stroke occurs primarily in young adults, may follow any route of administration, is frequently associated with vascular malformations, and presents with intracranial hemorrhage more commonly than with cerebral infarction.[13] *Young adults with stroke* require specialized etiologic investigation focusing on coagulopathies, antiphospholipid antibodies, ethanol intoxication, migraine, drug use, intimal dissection, patent foramen ovale, and human immunodeficiency virus (HIV).[14]

Risk-factor reduction through diet, exercise, cessation of smoking, and compliance with medical regimens is the most important preventive strategy in decreasing the incidence of stroke. The Systolic Hypertension in the Elderly Program (SHEP) found that in persons aged 60 years and over with isolated systolic hypertension, antihypertensive stepped-care drug treatment with low-dose chlorthalidone reduced the incidence of total stroke by 36 percent.[15] A Veterans Administration study of hypertensive men found that age and ethnic origin are important determinants of response to specific antihypertensive agents and recommended individualizing treatment based on these key demographic variables.[16] It must be recognized, however, that antihypertensive treatment can adversely affect perceived quality of life and possibly medication compliance.[17]

References

1. Grotta JC. Acute stroke management: Diagnosis. Stroke Clin Update III(5):17–24, 1993.

2. Chesebro JH, Fuster V, Halperin JL. Atrial fibrillation—Risk marker for stroke. N Engl J Med 323:1556–1558, 1990.

3. Abbott RD, Yin Y, Reed DM, et al. Risk of stroke in male cigarette smokers. N Engl J Med 315:717–720, 1986.

4. Olsen ML. Autoimmune disease and stroke. Stroke Clin Update III(4): 13–16, 1992.

5. Benjamin EJ, Plehn JF, D'Agostino RB. Mitral annular calcification and the risk of stroke in an elderly cohort. N Engl J Med 327:374–379, 1992.

6. Barnett HJM, Boughner DR, Taylor DW. Further evidence relating mitral-valve prolapse to cerebral ischemic events. N Engl J Med 302: 139–144, 1980.

7. Maggioni AP, Franzosi MG, Santoro E. The risk of stroke in patients with acute myocardial infarction after thrombolytic and antithrombotic treatment. N Engl J Med 327:1–6, 1992.

8. National Stroke Association. Stroke Facts at a Glance. Be Smart! Englewood, CO: NSA Brochure, 1993.

9. Kittner SJ, White LR, Losonczy KG, et al. Black–white differences in stroke incidence in a national sample. JAMA 264(10):1267–1270, 1990.

10. Broderick JP, Brott T, Tomsick T, et al. The risk of subarachnoid and intracerebral hemorrhages in blacks as compared to whites. N Engl J Med 326:733–736, 1992.

11. Klatsky AL, Armstrong MA, Friedman GD. Racial differences in cerebrovascular disease hospitalizations. Stroke 22:299–304, 1991.

12. Rowbotham MC. Neurologic aspects of cocaine abuse. West J Med 149: 442–448, 1988.

13. Klonoff DC, Andrews BT, Obana WG. Stroke associated with cocaine use. Arch Neurol 46:989–993, 1989.

14. Mitiguy J. Ischemic stroke in young adults: Conditions, behaviors, risks. Headlines 4:2–8, 1993.

15. SHEP Cooperative Research Group. Prevention of stroke by antihypertensive drug treatment in older persons with isolated systolic hypertension. JAMA 265:3255–3264, 1991.

16. Materson BJ, Reda DJ, Cushman WC, et al. Single-drug therapy for hypertension in men. N Engl J Med 328:914–921, 1993.

17. Testa MA, Anderson RB, Nackley JF, et al. Quality of life and antihypertensive therapy in men. N Engl J Med 328:907–913, 1993.

Suggested Reading

Be Stroke Smart. Englewood, CO: National Stroke Association Newsletter, quarterly.

A Guide for Weight Reduction. Dallas: American Heart Association, 1975.

Stroke: Reducing Your Risk. Englewood, CO: National Stroke Association, 1989.

What Is a Stroke? Chicago: American Association of Neurological Surgeons and Congress of Neurological Surgeons, 1990.

2

Initial Evaluation and Intervention

The treatment the stroke patient receives in the emergency, critical care, and medical–surgical departments of an acute-care hospital or trauma center sets the foundation for neurologic and functional recovery in rehabilitation. Different treatments are indicated for the various stroke syndromes, so it is imperative that an accurate diagnosis be made promptly. The National Stroke Association (NSA) recently circulated a consensus statement calling for aggressive, comprehensive treatment in the early stages of stroke.[1] Borrowing from the critical care model of cardiac ischemia, the consensus panel proposed a "brain attack" paradigm. Although an exhaustive discussion of acute management principles is beyond the scope of this book, a general discussion will facilitate the rehabilitation provider's understanding of the complex care the stroke victim experiences.

Initial treatment generally consists of history, physical examination, and neuroimaging.[2-5] Accompanying family and friends often provide the history as patients may be unable to respond to intensive inquiry. Questioning includes determination of the patient's age, time, and onset pattern of the event; evaluation of past medical history and risk factors for stroke—hypertension, cardiac dysrhythmia such as atrial fibrillation, diabetes mellitus, obesity, cigarette use, high blood

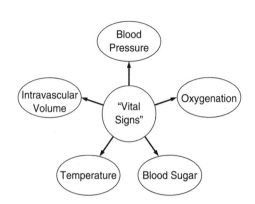

FIGURE 2.1 *Initial assessment and intervention in suspected stroke.*

(Adapted from Grotta J. Acute stroke management. Stroke Clin Update III:21, 1993. Used with permission of the National Stroke Association, Englewood, CO.)

lipid levels, prior neurologic illness, peripheral vascular disease, drug use, and recent trauma; and assessment of patient symptoms—weakness, lack of coordination, headache, drooling, mental status changes, numbness, tingling, gait problems, seizure activity, swallowing or breathing difficulty, visual change, dizziness, speech-language problems, and fatigue.

The directed emergency examination provides additional information to corroborate the diagnostic impression obtained from the history. Chemistry, hematology, and coagulation lab work are needed, as well as assessment of airway, breathing, circulation, and the cardiac function (Figure 2.1). The neurologic examination, while mandatory, may be brief and limited by the patient's ability to participate. Table 2.1 provides a lengthy outline of the components of mental status although only certain aspects may be assessed initially. A mental status examination determines a patient's level of alertness and consciousness, orientation, language ability, and cognitive capacity. The cranial nerve examination assesses the fundi (looking for papilledema as evidence of increased intracranial pressure); visual field and/or visuoperceptual deficits; facial weakness and sensory loss; oropharyngeal, lingual, and ocular paralysis; nystagmus; and olfactory and swallowing dysfunction.

Additional information as to the amount of limb weakness, tone, spasticity, and degree of proprioceptive, light touch, deep pressure, and hot/cold sense preservation comes from the motor and sensory examinations, which also aid in assessing cognition. The reflex examination demonstrates muscle stretch response, emergence of pathologic reflexes, and frontal release signs (such as glabellar, palmomental,

TABLE 2.1 Neurologic Examination

I. Mental Status:
Orientation (time, place, person); state of consciousness; information, memory, calculation, language function; special: aphasia, apraxia, agnosia

II. Cranial Nerves:
1. Smell
2. Fundi; visual fields, acuity
3,4,6. Pupils (direct, consensual), EOM movements, nystagmus
5. Sensation, corneals, jaw jerk, jaw movement
7. Facial movement: upper–lower; taste
8. Hearing (watch-tick; Weber, Rinne)
9,10. Gag reflex, palate movement
11. Sternocleidomastoid, trapezii
12. Tongue protrusion, power, fasciculations, dysarthria

III. Strength and Coordination
Ambulation: gait, station, heel, toe, hopping, tandem, Romberg
Motor Power: drift, direct muscle testing (hemiparesis, paraparesis, proximal weakness, distal weakness, radicular pattern, peripheral nerve pattern)
Tone: Spasticity, rigidity (axial, limb)
Coordination: Finger-finger-nose (F-F-N), rapid alternating movement (R-A-M), heel-knee-shin (H-K-S), heel tapping
Spontaneous Movement: Fasciculations, tremor, chorea, myoclonus, athetosis, dystonia, etc.

IV. Reflexes:
Deep Tendon Reflexes: biceps, triceps, knee, brachioradialis, ankle; Grade: 0–4
Superficial: abdominal, cremasteric
Plantar: Babinski, Chaddock, Oppenheim, Gordon
Frontal Lobe: suck, grasp
Corticobulbar: snout, palmar-mental
Meningeal: Kernig, Brudzinski

V. Sensation:
Primary: touch, pinprick, vibration, position (abnormal pattern: distal–symmetrical; dermatomal; isolated nerve)
Cortical: double simultaneous stimulation: extinction, adaptation; stereognosis; graphesthesia; point localization; face–hand

VI. Vascular: carotid pulses; bruits (carotid, subclavian arteries, eyes)

snout, root, grasp, and suck reflexes) and other indicators of cerebral function. The cerebellar examination appraises balance, coordination, and gait.

Coma is a special problem in some patients with focal stroke.[6] Defined as the absence of arousability or conscious awareness, *coma* may indicate damage to the reticular activating system, brain stem, bilateral hemispheres, or a combination. Coma in stroke typically bodes a poor prognosis for good recovery.

Sophisticated neuroimaging provides additional information to pinpoint the type and distribution of stroke. Computed tomography (CT) is widely available, well tolerated, and effectively differentiates infarct from hemorrhage. All stroke patients should receive an emergent noncontrast head CT to look for intracranial hemorrhage because CT readily demonstrates acute cerebral *hemorrhage*. Often acute cerebral *infarction* does not appear on the initial CT scan because it may take a few days for cellular damage to evolve demonstrably. A large infarction that produces prominent edema may be suspected on initial CT (Figures 2.2A, B).

Although more expensive and time-consuming, magnetic resonance imaging (MRI) better identifies gray and white matter changes and demonstrates ischemic stroke sooner than CT (Figures 2.3 and 2.4A, B). MRI rarely is indicated in the emergency evaluation of stroke. Acute subarachnoid hemorrhage easily can be missed with MRI and the seriously ill patient often cannot tolerate the procedure because of the confined space and length of the exam.

Specialized applications of MRI improve imaging speed, sensitivity, and usefulness. Magnetic resonance angiography (MRA) can demonstrate medium to large vessel occlusions outside the brain and in the base of the skull, arteriovenous malformations, and large aneurysms (Figure 2.5). Diffusion-weighted MRI uses rapidly changing magnetic fields to detect the surge of water that rushes through brain cells after injury thereby determining the severity and reversibility of cerebral ischemia. Echo planar imaging provides this information even more quickly. Perfusion MRI allows evaluation of cerebral perfusion at the capillary level.

Two radionuclide technologies provide important information about brain function. Single-photon-emission computed tomography (SPECT) is used to study cerebral blood flow, cerebral blood volume, and cerebral neurotransmitter receptors. Positron-emission tomography (PET) provides similar information with better spatial resolution, though at higher cost than SPECT. Although neither of these tech-

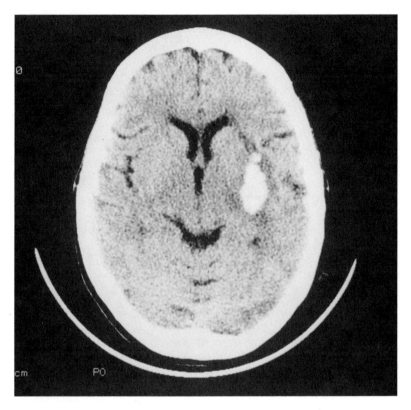

FIGURE 2.2A   *CT scan of the brain without contrast, demonstrating right basal ganglial hemorrhage.*

nologies is yet in widespread clinical use, they continue to play a role in the diagnosis and treatment of cerebral perfusion abnormalities.

The blood vessels of the head and neck also can be visualized by arteriography and ultrasonography. *Arteriography* involves intravascular injection of contrast material and is used to definitively diagnose arteriovenous malformation, aneurysm and dissection, and stenosis of intracranial and extracranial vessels. Even though this procedure is invasive, complications are few in competent hands. Doppler *ultrasonography* uses sound waves to image the carotid arteries. Although noninvasive, the technique significantly depends on the skill of the ultrasonographer and is most useful for screening for cervical internal carotid stenosis (Figure 2.6).[7] Where available, transcranial Doppler

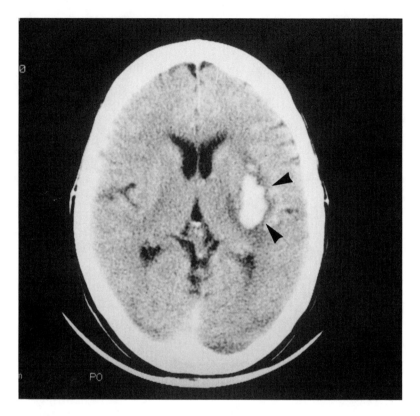

FIGURE 2.2B   *CT scan of the brain with contrast; surrounding edema enhanced with contrast.*

ultrasonography is used to assess blood flow particularly in the vertebral, basilar, distal carotid, and proximal middle cerebral arteries.

The lifesaving initial treatment often disorients and confuses the stroke victim. The hospital emergency room (ER) is foreign to most people. Curtains and visiting restrictions isolate patients from visual stimulation, friends, and families. The neuroimaging techniques, particularly MRI, can cause agitation, claustrophobia, and panic. Many patients have fearful memories of their emergency treatment that recur during rehabilitation.

Once the diagnosis has been accurately made, additional interventions may occur. Cerebral infarction treatment includes judicious blood pressure control; it is important not to aggressively lower the

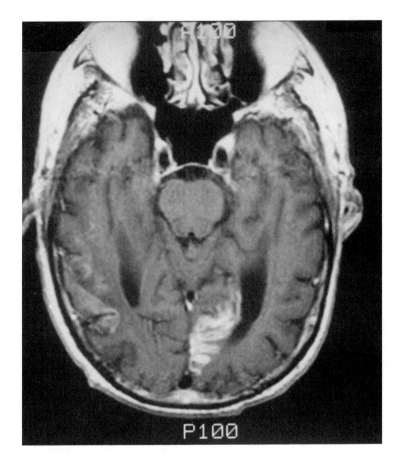

FIGURE 2.3   *MRI brain scan with gadolinium, demonstrating gyral enhancement in left occipital lobe.*

blood pressure because this may result in more extensive infarction.[8,9] Seizures require treatment with full doses of antiseizure medication, usually phenytoin. Thrombolytic therapy is gaining acceptance to acutely dissolve clots that compromise blood flow (Figure 2.7).

Surgical treatment of cerebrovascular disease continues to evolve. In 1988, Winslow published a critique of excessive carotid endarterectomy in which she notes a high-complication rate of 9.8 percent, prompting a barrage of public outcry and scientific studies designed to clarify the indications for this surgery.[10] Mayberg then found that men with significant carotid stenosis on the side appropriate to their

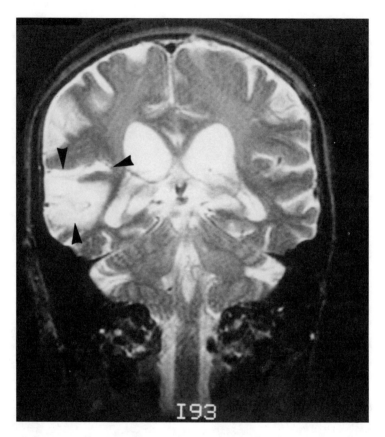

FIGURE 2.4A   *MRI of brain in coronal section without gadolinium contrast.*

symptoms safely and effectively reduced their risk of subsequent ipsilateral ischemia after carotid endarterectomy.[11] Carotid endarterectomy subsequently has proven beneficial for patients with recent transient ischemic attacks, hemispheric, or nondisabling strokes and ipsilateral high-grade stenosis.[12] In a study of 444 men, carotid endarterectomy for asymptomatic carotid stenosis did not significantly influence incidence of later stroke and death and cannot be definitely recommended for this condition.[13] Extracranial–intracranial arterial bypass does not appear to decrease the risk of ischemic strokes in patients who have symptomatic ischemia because of carotid and middle cerebral vascular disease.[14]

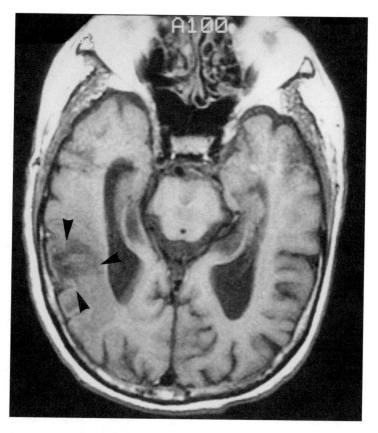

FIGURE 2.4B   *MRI of brain in transverse section with gadolinium contrast, demonstrating right posterior–temporal ischemia.*

Subarachnoid hemorrhage because of aneurysmal rupture is potentially life-threatening. Patients need neurosurgical consultation, blood pressure correction, calcium channel blockade (to prevent vasospasm), aggressive treatment of seizures, and hemodynamic and intracerebral pressure monitoring. Diuretics such as mannitol, intubation, and mechanical ventilation may be needed to decrease intracranial pressure. Once the aneurysm is identified on angiography, the patient may undergo emergent aneurysmal clipping or resection. The patient may also require ventriculoperitoneal shunt placement for treatment of obstructive hydrocephalus (secondary to cerebrospinal fluid accu-

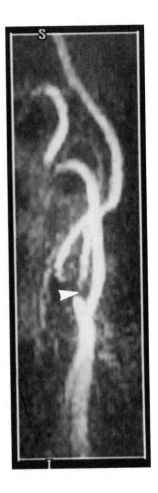

FIGURE 2.5 *MRA demonstrating 99 percent stenosis/near occlusion of right internal carotid artery.*

mulation in any of the brain's ventricles), which may occur when the arachnoid granulations become clogged by blood, thus preventing resorption of cerebrospinal fluid (CSF).

Intraparenchymal cerebral hemorrhage carries an extremely high incidence of morbidity and mortality. Extremely high blood pressure requires correction, as does high intracranial pressure. Early surgical evacuation of moderate- to large-size cerebral hematomas in conscious patients may be performed. Cerebellar infarction requires neurosurgical consultation for possible decompression; with large hemorrhage or infarctions, brainstem compression is likely, and there is an urgent need for surgical removal, even in patients with coma.

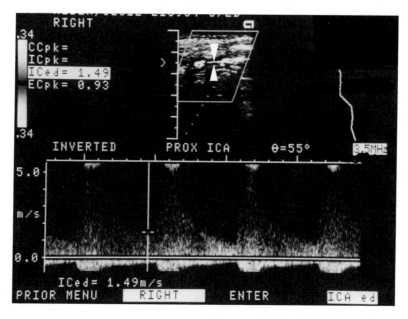

FIGURE 2.6 *Duplex Doppler sonogram demonstrating 99 percent stenosis/near occlusion of right internal carotid artery.*

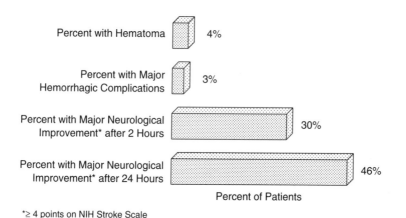

Percent with Hematoma — 4%

Percent with Major Hemorrhagic Complications — 3%

Percent with Major Neurological Improvement* after 2 Hours — 30%

Percent with Major Neurological Improvement* after 24 Hours — 46%

Percent of Patients

*≥ 4 points on NIH Stroke Scale

FIGURE 2.7 *Thrombolytic therapy in stroke.*

(Adapted from Stroke Clin Update III:23, 1992. Used with permission of the National Stroke Association, Englewood, CO.)

Antiplatelet treatment with aspirin or ticlopidine or full anticoagulation with heparin or warfarin may be begun in patients with ischemic stroke (Table 2.2).[15] Newer recommendations incorporate age and cardiac risk factors in antithrombotic therapy (Table 2.3). In patients with intolerance to aspirin or who experience stroke warnings while on aspirin, ticlopidine is a proven alternative for prevention.[16] Additionally, women, patients with vertebrobasilar symptoms, and patients with diffuse atherosclerotic disease tolerate ticlopidine better than aspirin.[17] Anticoagulation with heparin is considered in progressing stroke, recent TIA, and cardioembolic stroke.[18] Some practitioners prefer to wait 48 hours after stroke to begin heparin because of concern about a hemorrhagic transformation. Long-term low-dose warfarin therapy is highly effective and generally safe in preventing stroke in patients with nonrheumatic atrial fibrillation.[19-21] The stroke survivor and family may voice uncertainty about secondary stroke prevention. The rehabilitation provider can take every opportunity to educate the family and patient and help reduce the risk of stroke recurrence.[22]

TABLE 2.2   Antiplatelet Treatment in Ischemic Stroke

ASA/Ticlopidine	Primary prevention of stroke for males older than 50 with stroke risk factors
	Primary prevention when atherosclerotic cerebrovascular disease present
	Asymptomatic carotid disease
	Symptomatic carotid disease less than 70% stenosis
	Transient ischemic attack
	Secondary prevention of stroke
	? vertebrobasilar ischemia
Carotid Endarterectomy	Symptomatic carotid stenosis greater than 70%
	? for asymptomatic carotid disease
Warfarin*	Primary prevention of stroke in patients with nonrheumatic atrial fibrillation
	Treatment and secondary prevention of cardioembolic stroke

*The utility of warfarin is clarified in Table 2.3.

TABLE 2.3 Effect of Age and Cardiac Risk Factors on Antithrombotic Therapy

Age	No Risk Factors/Lone AF	Risk Factors Present
Younger than 60	No medication	Warfarin
60–75	Aspirin	Warfarin
Older than 75	Warfarin	Warfarin

Note: Risk factors include hypertension, prior stroke or TIA, diabetes mellitus, coronary artery disease, and congestive heart failure.

The acute management of the stroke patient is complicated and constantly evolving. Prognostication as to long-term survival and functional outcome is notoriously inaccurate in the intensive care setting. The myriad of treatment options may confuse patients and their families resulting in uncertainty, anxiety, depression, and delayed neurologic and functional recovery. Many patients only begin to realize the extent of their acute-care hospital treatment after they enter rehabilitation. Rehabilitation providers need to familiarize themselves with acute medical and surgical management of stroke so that they can ease stroke patients' processing of their recent experiences. Support and understanding by rehabilitation caregivers can do much to improve long-term stroke recovery.

References

1. McDowell FH. Stroke: The first six hours. National Stroke Association Consensus Statement. Stroke Clin Update IV:1–12, 1993.

2. Grotta JC. Acute stroke management (in three parts). Stroke Clin Update III:17–24, 1992, and IV:13–16, 1993.

3. Gilman S. Advances in neurology. N Engl J Med 326:1608–1616, 1671–1676, 1992.

4. Grotta JC. Current medical and surgical therapy for cerebrovascular disease. N Engl J Med 317:1505–1516, 1987.

5. Caplan LR. Diagnosis and treatment of ischemic stroke. JAMA 266:2413–2418, 1991.

6. Frank JI, Biller J. Coma in focal cerebrovascular disease: An overview. Stroke Clin Update III:9–12, 1992.

7. Latchaw RE. Imaging the patient with ischemic cerebrovascular disease. Stroke Clin Update II:13–16, 1991.

8. Yatsu FM, Zivin J. Hypertension in acute ischemic strokes. Arch Neurol 42:999–1002, 1985.

9. Fletcher AE, Bulpitt CJ. How far should blood pressure be lowered? N Engl J Med 326:251–254, 1992.

10. Winslow CM, Solomon DH, Chassin MR. The appropriateness of carotid endarterectomy. N Engl J Med 318:721–727, 1988.

11. Mayberg MR, Wilson SE, Yatsu F, et al. Carotid endarterectomy and prevention of cerebral ischemia in symptomatic carotid stenosis. JAMA 266:3289–3294, 1991.

12. Neville RF, Hobson RW. Indications for carotid endarterectomy: An update. Stroke Clin Update II:5–8, 1991.

13. Hobson RWM, Weiss DG, Fields WS, et al. Efficacy of carotid endarterectomy for asymptomatic carotid stenosis. N Engl J Med 328: 221–227, 1993.

14. The EC/IC Bypass Study Group. Failure of extracranial-intracranial arterial byass to reduce the risk of ischemic stroke. N Engl J Med 313: 1191–1200, 1985.

15. Goodnight SH, Coull BM, McAnulty JH, et al. Antiplatelet therapy. West J Med 158:385–392, 506–514, 1993.

16. Hass W. Ticlopidine: An antiplatelet drug useful in stroke prevention. Stroke Clin Update II:21–24, 1992.

17. Grotta JC, Norris JW, Kamm B. Prevention of stroke with ticlopidine: Who benefits most? Neurology 42:111–115, 1992.

18. Miller VT, Hart RG. Heparin anticoagulation in acute brain ischemia. Stroke 19:403–406, 1988.

19. The Boston Area Anticoagulation Trial for Atrial Fibrillation. The effect of low-dose warfarin on the risk of stroke in patients with nonrheumatic atrial fibrillation. N Engl J Med 323:1505–1511, 1990.

20. Ezekowitz MD, Bridgers SL, James KE, et al. Warfarin in the prevention of stroke associated with nonrheumatic atrial fibrillation. N Engl J Med 327:1406–1412, 1992.

21. Singer DE. Randomized trials of warfarin for atrial fibrillation. N Engl J Med 327:1451–1453, 1992.

22. Goldberg G, Berger GG. Secondary prevention in stroke: A primary rehabilitation concern. Arch Phys Med Rehabil 69:32–40, 1988.

3

Medical Complications
of Stroke

Prevention and early recognition of medical complications of stroke best maximizes neurologic and functional recovery. Development of these problems may precipitate major setbacks in the process of functional recovery, offset the gains accomplished through comprehensive rehabilitation following stroke, raise rates of rehospitalization and increase health-care costs.[1,2] Chapter 11 discusses the effect of medical complications on functional outcome and restoration. All rehabilitation providers have the opportunity to recognize signs and symptoms of these impediments to recovery. This chapter discusses ways to prevent and assess secondary complications after stroke.

Thromboembolic Disease

Deep venous thrombosis (DVT) and pulmonary embolism (PE) are frequent complications after stroke.[3,4] A *deep venous thrombosis* is a clot in the deep veins of the leg. This may cause unilateral leg swelling, superficial venous prominence, pain in the affected leg particularly with ankle dorsiflexion, redness of involved extremity, tenderness to palpation, and other symptoms. Left untreated, this clot may break off from the venous intima and travel to the pulmonary vasculature, causing a PE. Pulmonary embolism typically presents with sudden onset of *dyspnea* (shortness of breath and difficulty breathing), *pleuritic* chest pain (sharp, stabbing chest pain more pronounced with a deep breath), and hypoxemia. Hypoxemia may lead to a change in skin color, confusion, frank change in consciousness, or unresponsiveness. Signs and symptoms of PE may also be more subtle and require a high degree of clinical vigilance.

The reported incidence of DVT after stroke is 40% to 50% and of PE is 9% to 15%. These thromboembolic phenomena are the fourth most common cause of death in the first 30 days after stroke. The time of greatest risk is 4 to 5 days after stroke which is often when mobilization efforts begin, though the period of high risk extends up to three months after stroke. Classic predisposing factors include *venous stasis* (pooling of blood because of immobility), *hypercoagulability* (tendency to clot more readily than normal), and venous wall lining (*endothelial*) injury. The acute stroke patient usually is immobilized and may have increased coagulability because of release of systemic factors after intracerebral damage, so generally has at least two risk factors.

Because of the high risk of thromboembolic disease after a stroke, prevention of these problems is of paramount importance. Patients with bland (nonhemorrhagic) stroke should receive subcutaneous heparin as prophylaxis; the appropriate frequency and duration of such treatment remains unclear. It is common for patients to receive 5000 units of heparin subcutaneously every 12 hours until they can walk unassisted or until rehabilitation discharge. Patients with hemorrhagic stroke may be at increased risk for additional bleeding if placed on heparin within the first 7 to 14 days after stroke; options for early prevention include placement of a blood filter in the inferior vena cava or intermittent pneumatic compression of the legs.

Recognition of DVT is difficult. Perhaps 50 percent of important DVTs are not clinically apparent. Noninvasive testing, including Doppler ultrasonography and fibrinogen scanning, accurately screen and diagnose the vast majority of thrombi, although even those are clinically silent. Recommendations for use of these modalities vary widely; however, it is not uncommon to see regular (on admission, every two weeks during hospitalization, and at discharge) Doppler testing. Additionally, it is wise to obtain a baseline oxygen saturation for stroke patients so that any change that might be attributable to PE can be compared with a baseline value.

The rehabilitation provider can facilitate prophylaxis by mobilizing the patient as quickly as the patient's clinical condition allows; ambulation decreases risk of DVT and PE. Other forms of mobilization (lower-extremity resistive exercise and standing) may alter risk, but this is not known with certainty. Because so many of these clots are difficult to recognize, all caregivers should maintain a high index of suspicion for thromboembolic phenomena throughout the rehabilitation process and should be aware of any change in the lower-extremity exam. If PE is suspected, testing, such as ventilation/perfusion scanning or pulmonary angiography, can be performed quickly and proper therapy instituted as indicated.

Even though heparin prophylaxis does not result in full, systemic anticoagulation, the patient may have an increased propensity to hemorrhage. Care should be taken to avoid blunt trauma, falling, or other injuries that can cause hematoma formation in damaged tissues. Hematuria, especially with concomitant Foley catheter use or occult blood in stool, may develop in patients on subcutaneous heparin. A "bleeding precautions" system like the one shown in Table 3.1 can be used to alert all rehabilitation providers to those patients receiving prophylactic and systemic anticoagulants.

Respiratory Complications

Pneumonia, an acute infection of the alveolar spaces of the lung, may involve an entire lung lobe, certain segments, and/or the alveoli adjacent to the bronchus.[5] The incidence of pneumonia with all types of strokes is 32%, but is higher with subarachnoid hemorrhage and patients with coma. Pneumonia is the third major cause of death in the first 30 days after a stroke and causes 7% to 34% of deaths in stroke patients. Common risk factors for pneumonia include aspiration of oral contents including saliva, liquids, and food; decreased chest wall compliance; poor expiratory muscle strength so that forced coughing is impaired; depressed immune response after stroke; and general debility. Classically, onset is sudden with shaking chills, pleuritic pain on the involved side, cough with sputum production, fever, headache, nausea, and vomiting. In stroke patients, pneumonia may be difficult to recognize, presenting only with a low-grade fever, lethargy, loss of neurologic or functional status, and malaise. The rehabilitation provider should be alert for these findings, because prompt diagnosis and treatment of

TABLE 3.1   Bleeding Precautions Developed by the Nursing Department
at The Rehabilitation Institute at Santa Barbara

I. **Policy:**
Patients who are on anticoagulation therapy or have a medical condition (i.e., blood dyscrasias such as thrombocytopenia), which may increase their risk of prolonged bleeding, will be placed on bleeding precautions.

II. **Purpose:**
To ensure patients' safety during anticoagulation therapy and when medical conditions warrant extra measures to watch for and prevent excessive bleeding.

III. **Equipment:**
Side rails, pads; electric razor; soft toothbrush

IV. **Procedure:**
1. Before administering an anticoagulant, the nurse is required to refer to the most current lab result and review the PT or PTT value. When documenting dosage administered, the nurse should record this value directly under his or her initials on the Medication Administration Record (MAR).
2. If the patient has an anticoagulant ordered and no current lab result is available (i.e., on the first hospital day), communication with the physician must take place to determine if the referring hospital has lab data available. This communication must be documented on the nurse's progress notes and Kardex so current lab data can be available to all staff.
3. Observe for bleeding (e.g., in the stool, urine, nose, vagina, gum, or as indicated by any abnormal bruising or petechiae). Check urine and stools for OB daily.
4. Protect patients from trauma. Keep side rails up and pad side rails if indicated. Use electric razor. Use soft toothbrush and gentle oral care, remove dentures if necessary. Avoid use of adhesive tape. Lubricate lips and protect all skin surfaces.
5. Limit venipunctures. If venipuncture is absolutely necessary, apply pressure for 20 minutes.
6. No intramuscular injections. If absolutely necessary, use z-track technique.
7. Avoid constipation and straining to have a bowel movement. Digital stimulation should be done gently to avoid irritation of mucosa. Encourage soft, bland nonirritating diet.
8. Avoid prolonged inflation of cuff during blood pressure checks and rotate extremities to avoid bruising.
9. Check platelet count daily when indicated.

pneumonia with intravenous fluids, antibiotics, and tracheobronchial hygiene improves the chances of survival. Encouragement of deep breathing and forced expiration at regular intervals can prevent atelectasis that may predispose stroke patients to pneumonia.

Other respiratory problems include alteration in the normal breathing mechanism. Many patients hyperventilate after stroke, especially those with severely impaired motor control. This is a poor prognostic sign because it indicates damage to the respiratory motor-control area of the brain. Another alteration in breathing, Cheyne-Stokes pattern, may be seen, particularly in patients with concomitant heart or renal disease. In general, significant alterations in an acute stroke patient's breathing pattern evidences a large area of brain damage or brainstem dysfunction.

Over the long term, the stroke survivor may experience other changes in breathing. As spasticity and chest wall contracture develop after stroke, the patient may have decreased chest movement on the weak side, decreased chest wall compliance, and poor motor control of inspiration and expiration. These problems are compounded by persistence of inspiratory and expiratory muscle weakness, which limits thoracic excursion and intercostal muscle functioning. The end result may be restrictive pulmonary dysfunction. The rehabilitation provider should focus on flexibility and strength development in an effort to alleviate these problems and needs to develop a daily regimen for the patient to follow.

Cardiac Disease

Most patients suffer a stroke because of some type of vascular disease. It is reasonable to assume that these patients have disease affecting other blood vessels as well, particularly those that supply the heart. At least 75% of stroke patients have cardiac disease, which may have caused the stroke, and may impact stroke recovery.[6] Cardiac disease is the second leading cause of early mortality and the leading cause of late mortality after stroke. Of stroke patients, 66% have coronary artery disease, 50% have dysrhythmias, and 20% have congestive heart failure.

Many different types of cardiac problems can cause stroke. *Atrial fibrillation,* an arrhythmia that results from the continuous and chaotic reentry of electrical impulses within the atria causing fragmentary and ineffective atrial contraction, can precipitate emboli that travel to the cerebral circulation. Atrial fibrillation usually is caused by rheumatic heart disease or atherosclerotic cardiovascular disease; it may occur intermittently, particularly with cardiac strain, or continuously. Other dysrhythmias, anatomic variations, or myocardial infarctions may precipitate formation of clots in the heart that may dislodge causing embolic stroke. Cardiac valvular vegetations, classically seen in bacterial endocarditis, may develop as a result of systemic infections. These can also embolize to the cerebral vessels, leading to stroke. In shock from myocardial infarction, trauma, systemic infection, immune dysfunction, or other diseases, the heart may not pump as intended, resulting in systemic hypotension. The decrease in perfusion limits brain oxygenation causing stroke, particularly in the watershed areas of the brain that are most prone to loss of blood flow.

Moreover, heart dysfunction can also be caused by stroke. Ventricular dysrhythmia is often seen with subarachnoid hemorrhage. Stroke appears to cause loss of neural cardioregulation and release of transmitters that stimulate cardiac electrical conduction. To more fully define the relationship between the neurologic and cardiovascular systems, research in cardioneurology is ongoing.

Most commonly, cardiovascular and neurovascular disease is seen concomitantly. A study of 38 patients with completed stroke found that 60 percent of them showed coronary artery disease on dipyridamole stress testing. Unfortunately, many measures of cardiac work are not standardized to the population in rehabilitation. One has difficulty knowing how much activity and exercise a given stroke patient's cardiovascular system can tolerate because almost all studies of cardiac performance have been done with physically able people.

Generally, it is safe to assume all elderly stroke patients have some significant cardiovascular disease. At The Rehabilitation Institute at Santa Barbara, we monitor blood pressure daily with peak exercise; question patients frequently as to fatigue, chest discomfort, and feeling of well-being; and include answers to these inquiries on the communication boards for the language impaired. We use telemetry, monitored by nurses trained in dysrhythmia recognition, to assess patients during exercise. Although exercise prescription cannot be accurately guided by standard measures of metabolic equivalency, these steps have been useful in limiting cardiac morbidity and mortality.

Some cardiac disease may not be discovered until the patient is subjected to the stress of exercise. Vigorous monitoring of pulse, blood pressure, and exercise tolerance during rehabilitation may identify signs of cardiac dysfunction. If found, appropriate investigation for disturbances in cardiac rhythm, perfusion, and function can be undertaken.

Neurologic Change

Seizures complicate less than 10 percent of all strokes.[7,8] Half occur in the first few days after stroke. Later seizures are seen more commonly in patients with embolic or hemorrhagic stroke and in those who have been comatose. *Seizure,* a disorder of cerebral electrical activities, can result in altered consciousness, abnormal movement or sensation, or inappropriate behavior. In seizure after stroke, the neurologic presentation typically parallels the function of the infarcted brain. *Partial* seizures are those in which a focal or localized onset can be discerned and *generalized* seizures are those that involve both sides of the brain. Partial seizures may be *simple* (without alteration in consciousness) such as simple tonic, clonic, tonic–clonic, or sensory seizures or *complex* (with impairment in consciousness) such as complex partial seizures. Generalized seizures may be tonic, clonic, tonic–clonic (grand mal), or absence (petit mal). Other less common seizure types are rarely seen after stroke and are not discussed here.

The rehabilitation therapist may be the first to witness post-stroke seizures, because they may occur more commonly in settings of physical fatigue and emotional stress. *Motor* seizures (convulsions) generally are apparent because of generalized extension or simple movement of specific body parts. Many patients have an *aura*—an unnatural, remembered experience—prior to the actual seizure. Petit mal seizures are notable for their lack of motor involvement and present with interruption of consciousness. Sometimes only a loss of the conversation or place in the performance of a task belies the seizure occurrence.

Assessment of seizure usually includes electroencephalograph (EEG) and other neurologic testing. In this procedure, surface electrodes are placed on the scalp to monitor brain activity. Sleep deprivation, photic stimulation, and other maneuvers may be performed to enhance the sensitivity of EEG. The patient may find this test fatiguing. EEG helps to a varying extent in specific localization of seizure focus after stroke.

Patients with post-stroke seizure are routinely treated with antiseizure medications such as phenytoin, phenobarbital, carbamazepine, valproic acid, and so forth. Although controversial, some patients at risk for seizure after stroke may be given preventive antiseizure medication even without having had an actual seizure. All antiseizure medications impair cognition to some extent; there is no evidence of a marked side-effect advantage of any one preparation. A "seizure precautions" communication system to alert therapists and staff of potential or actual seizure and use of antiseizure medication is useful in stroke rehabilitation (see Appendix). Treatment plans and expectations can then be modified with these parameters in mind.

Bowel and Bladder Dysfunction

Most stroke patients have some dysfunction of bowel and bladder, which usually begins early in the hospital course.[9-12] Bladder continence is a complex feat of awareness, control, mobility, and dexterity and is vulnerable at many points to the direct and indirect effects of cerebrovascular disease. Site, size, number of strokes, time elapsed since stroke, voiding history, motor function, depression, patients' expectations, and urogenitary disease affect continence. Acute stroke of any type can cause brainstem dysfunction and resultant incontinence. Cortical lesions can give symptoms of urinary urgency at low urine volumes and urine incontinence because of an unstable detrusor, the most common cystometric finding in stroke survivors with moderate or severe persistent incontinence. Brainstem strokes below the pons can cause detrusor/sphincter dyssynergia. Large strokes, especially those resulting in aphasia, use of restraints, depression, and alteration in consciousness and cognition contribute to incontinence. Moreover, fecal impaction, pelvic floor weakness, and outlet obstruction commonly impact post-stroke bladder function.

Routinely, an indwelling catheter is placed at the acute-care hospital to facilitate fluid management and prevent skin breakdown and other problems of incontinence. At some point, the risks of continued catheter use, the most important being urinary tract infection, outweigh the inconvenience associated with removal of the device. At most institutions, catheters are removed based on the patient's functional status (particularly with achievement of moderately assisted transfers and fair balance), urologic health (prostate disease, micropenis), patient/family request, and assessed ability to participate in bladder retraining. Alternate periods of clamping and draining an indwelling catheter does not train a post-stroke bladder and has no role in stroke rehabilitation. Team management of incontinence minimizes staff discord and should emphasize behavioral modification; drug therapy and surgical intervention can follow. Fluid intake should be 1500 to 1800 ml in all forms over a 24-hour period. Bladder charting should completely record fluid intake, voided urinary volumes, and incontinent events for three consecutive days. Ultrasonographic evaluation of postvoid bladder volume is useful; two consecutive residual urines of greater than 150 ml suggest incomplete emptying, requiring pharmacologic intervention and sometimes urologic consultation. Table 3.2 lists medication options for treating bladder dysfunction.

For patients requiring more than moderate assistance in transfers, catheterization is preferred. Indwelling catheters are safe and effective, but predispose a patient to infection. An external catheter can be used for men with unstable bladders without urinary retention. With any type of catheter used for men, special care must be taken to prevent *phimosis*—swelling of foreskin because of prolonged retraction behind glans.

Training must follow a schedule of voiding, regardless of sensation of bladder fullness, every 2 to 4 hours. The patient should be directed to void preventively before the sensation threshold is reached. More specific direction may be needed for cognitively impaired patients. Distraction techniques, pelvic floor strengthening exercises, and biofeedback with use of auditory and visual cues can be effective in teaching continence. Biofeedback does not alter the physiologic parameters of the bladder.

Urinary tract infection after stroke occurs in most all patients. Usually these infections are transient and respond well to oral antibiotics.

Incontinence rates drop in the first three months after stroke. Fourteen percent of long-term geriatric survivors of stroke are incontinent, a figure comparable to that for the elderly population at large. The patient who was incontinent before stroke does not necessarily need to be incontinent after stroke.

Urinary retention also may occur after stroke. Treatment includes mobility training, appropriate bowel care, eliminating medications that cause retention, testing for pelvic outlet obstruction, pharmacologic intervention, and intermittent catheterization.

Bowel dysfunction after stroke is common because of physical inactivity, inadequate fluid and/or dietary fiber, psychologic disturbances, actual impact of neurologic lesion on central defecation centers, side effects of medication or dietary supplements, bowel infection, or impaction of the intestine by prolonged constipation. Stroke patients often have difficulty calling attention to their bowel needs or transferring to the commode. Bedpans, while useful, do not allow easy

TABLE 3.2   Medication Options for Bladder Dysfunction after Stroke

Medication	Mechanism of Action	Indication
Oxybutynin (Ditropan) up to 5 mg qid	Relaxes detrussor; internal sphincter tone	Control urge, incontinence, or frequent voiding
Imipramine (Tofranil) up to 100 mg qhs	Increases internal sphincter tone; central effects; decreases detrussor contractibility	Control urge, incontinence, or enuresis
Bethanechol (Urecholine) up to 50 mg qid	Increases detrussor contractibility	Facilitate complete emptying
Prazosin (Minipress) Terazosin (Hytrin)	Alpha blockade of external sphincter resulting in decreased tone	Decreases outlet obstruction and external sphincter dysfunction
Hyoscyamine (Levsin, Levsin/SL, or Levsinex)	Increases internal sphincter tone; decreases detrussor contractibility	Control urge, incontinence

defecation because of the loss of gravity assistance, embarrassment, and the unnatural position associated with their use. Many post-stroke patients develop significant consequences of bowel neglect including diarrhea, constipation, impaction, and pain and discomfort with defecation. Many people are very focused on frequency and size of routine bowel movements, which makes problems with defecation emotionally troubling.

Treatment of the dysfunctional bowel after stroke begins with an assessment of premorbid bowel habits. Proper fluid, nutrition, and dietary fiber must be restored. Patients should be encouraged to defecate in their normal position, if possible, given physical limitations. A program to enhance evacuation (using suppositories, laxatives, enemas, or combinations thereof) should start at admission and continue as needed. Enemas and suppositories, while messy, are more predictable than oral laxatives, which may result in defecation over a broad time frame. If laxatives are chosen, mineral oil should be avoided because of concern about vitamin malabsorption and pneumonitis. All rehabilitation providers should have a sense of the patient's bowel regimen so that cumbersome and embarrassing accidents can be avoided.

The basic goals of post-stroke toilet training are to prevent complications of bladder and bowel dysfunction and to preserve continence. Treatment should be planned so there is adequate duration and frequency of toileting. A routine schedule for urination should be developed for the recovering stroke patient, one that takes into account fluid intake, premorbid toileting habits, and medical issues such as use of diuretics and any concurrent urinary tract infection. The gastro-colic reflex causes the urge to defecate soon after meal(s).

The rehabilitation staff must work around the patient's bladder and bowel, not the other way around. Those who treat patients after eating should be prepared for the patients' potential need to have a bowel movement. At any institution, it is best to have all rehabilitation caregivers assist regularly with toileting. The more all staff assist patients in the toileting process, the less potential there is for patient embarrassment and staff conflict.

Pain

Pain is common after stroke.[13] Table 3.3 indicates common types of pain to expect following stroke and some treatment options. Despite the general bias, central pain after stroke is quite uncommon and may be due more to peripheral mechanisms of spasticity and contracture than to brain injury. Reflex sympathetic dystrophy (RSD)—referred to by some as shoulder–hand syndrome or complex regional pain syndrome, type I—presents classically with pain in the extremity associated with edema, dystrophic skin, and vasomotor instability.[14] Metacarpal-phalangeal tenderness in this context is a sensitive clinical sign of RSD. Triple-phase radionuclide bone scanning complemented by diagnostic and therapeutic sympathetic blockade confirm the diagnosis.[15] Shoulder pain because of subluxation, loss of range of motion, spasticity, and/or intrinsic shoulder pathology is not necessarily sympathetically mediated.[16] Although less common, lower-extremity pain may occur and result from vascular phenomena, hip fracture, (osteo)arthritis, genu recurvatum, bracing, and foot problems. Spasticity can cause significant pain and requires a comprehensive management approach (see Chapter 4).

Pain perception and response may be influenced by aphasia, alteration in sensation, other medical conditions, depression, and anxiety. Pain adds to the burden of stroke disability and may retard recovery.

TABLE 3.3   Pain in the Hemiplegic Arm Following Stroke

Shoulder–hand syndrome	Hand and forearm pain
Shoulder pain	Hand and wrist contractures
Shoulder contracture	Wrist fracture
Glenohumeral subluxation	Peripheral nerve entrapment
Humeral fracture	Brachial plexus neuropathy
Rotator cuff disorder	Central pain states
Bicipital tendinitis	
Acromioclavicular joint disorder	

(Adapted from Teasell RW (ed), Physical Medicine and Rehabilitation: State-of-the-Art Reviews, vol 7, p 134, 1993.)

Although few patients treated for pain after stroke gain complete analgesia, many are partly helped by coordinated, logical treatment.

Skin Troubles

The body's largest organ is often compromised after stroke. As skin ages, it becomes thinner and somewhat less resilient. Seemingly minor trauma can result in large skin tears. Patients who take corticosteroids have particularly delicate skin that can be easily injured. Immobility, insensitivity, pressure, moisture, infection, incontinence, and nutritional deficiency are risk factors for development of skin breakdown after stroke.[17] Direct pressure, whether from shearing or weight bearing in sitting or recumbency, causes decubitus formation in about 15 percent of stroke patients. Treatment begins with prevention. A thin egg-crate mattress provides some relief from shearing forces; a thicker mattress may raise the bed too high, causing difficulty in transfer training. Highly sophisticated low or high air loss beds are not routinely indicated in preventative skin protection.

Once skin trouble develops, options for treatment abound. Some general principles are:

1. Avoid or dissipate pressure over the affected area using positioning techniques, pillow, and other cushioning.

2. Debride eschar and necrotic tissue sharply and/or with enzymatic cleansers.

3. Provide a healthy, protected area for healing to occur.

4. Monitor skin breakdown weekly with the skin care treatment team (physician, nurse-consultant, primary nurse, and physical therapist).

Currently, keeping the healing area moist with hydrophilic products, rather than using drying dressings, is recommended. Although povidone-iodine, hydrogen peroxide, and other bacteriostatic products may be used initially, avoid long-term (more than three days) use because these products can inhibit fibroblast production and may damage healthy granulating tissue.

Conclusion

Aggressive evaluation and management of medical complications after stroke appear to facilitate stroke recovery. The rehabilitation provider has the opportunity to recognize the signs and symptoms of these obstacles to improvement. Potentially, all organ systems can be adversely affected after stroke. Prompt recognition and diagnosis of medical problems improve patient care and outcome.

References

1. Moskowitz E. Complications in the rehabilitation of hemiplegic patients. Med Clin North Am 53:541–559, 1969.

2. Roth EJ. Medical complications encountered in stroke rehabilitation. In: Goldberg G (ed), Stroke Rehabilitation. Physical Medicine and Rehabilitation Clinics of North America, vol 2 (pp 563–578), 1991.

3. Warlow C, Ogston D, Douglas AS. Deep venous thrombosis of the legs and after strokes. BMJ 1:1178–1183, 1976.

4. Brandstater ME, Roth EJ, Siebens HC. Venous thromboembolism in stroke: Literature review and implications for clinical practice. Arch Phys Med Rehabil 73(suppl):379–391, 1992.

5. Scherzer HH, Nurse BA. Pneumonia in the elderly stroke patient. In: Erickson (ed), Medical Management of the Elderly Stroke Patient. Physical Medicine and Rehabilitation: State-of-the-Art Reviews, vol 3 (pp 519–536), 1989.

6. Roth EJ. Heart disease in patients with stroke. Arch Phys Med Rehabil 74:752–60; and 75:94–101, 1993.

7. Wiebe-Velazquez S, Blume WT. Seizures. In: Teasell RW (ed), Long-term Consequences of Stroke. Physical Medicine and Rehabilitation: State-of-the-Art Reviews, vol 7 (pp 73–87), 1993.

8. Olsen TS, Hogenhaven H, Thage O. Epilepsy after stroke. Neurology 37:1209–1211, 1987.

9. Currie CT. Urinary incontinence after stroke. BMJ 293:1322–1323, 1986.

10. Sedarat SM, Hecht JS. Urologic problems after stroke. Stroke Clin Update IV:17–25, 1993.

11. Borris MJ, Campbell AJ, Caradoc-Davies TH, et al. Urinary incontinence after stroke: A prospective study. Age Ageing 15:177–181, 1986.

12. Hoogasian S, Walzak MP, Wurzel R. Urinary incontinence in the stroke patient: Etiology and rehabilitation. In: Erickson (ed), Medical Management of the Elderly Stroke Patient. Physical Medicine and Rehabilitation: State-of-the-Art Reviews, vol 3 (pp 581–594), 1989.

13. Teasell RW. Pain following stroke. Critical Reviews in Physical and Rehabilitation Medicine, vol 3 (pp 205–217), 1992.

14. Davis SW, Petrillo CR, Eichberg RD, et al. Shoulder–hand syndrome in a hemiplegic population: A 5-year retrospective study. Arch Phys Med Rehabil 58:353–356, 1977.

15. Weiss L, Alfano A, Bardfeld P, et al. Prognostic value of triple phase bone scanning for reflex sympathetic dystrophy in hemiplegia. Arch Phys Med Rehabil 74:716–719, 1993.

16. Totta M, Beneck S. Shoulder dysfunction in stroke hemiplegia. Phys Med Rehabil Clin North Am 2:627–641, 1991.

17. Panel for the Prediction and Prevention of Pressure Ulcers in Adults. Pressure ulcers in adults: Prediction and prevention. Clinical Practice Guidelines, Number 3 (AHCPR Pub. No. 92-0047). Rockville, MD: Agency for Health Care Policy and Research, Public Health Service, U.S. Department of Health and Human Services, May 1992.

APPENDIX

Precautions for Care of Patient with Seizure

I. **Policy:**
The nurse is responsible for:
- Obtaining a seizure history and documenting it on admission
- Administering anticonvulsant medications per physician's orders and notifying the physician when problems with administration or schedule disruptions occur
- Recognizing patients at risk for seizures and instituting safety measures

II. **Purpose:**
To identify high-risk patients and to describe preventive interventions that promote patient safety and accurate assessment and contribute to the diagnosis of a seizure disorder.

III. **Equipment:**
   A. Padded side-rail protectors or cotton blankets and tape
   B. Oral airway
   C. Crash cart
   D. "Seizure precaution" signs

IV. **Essential Steps:**
   A. Identification and preventive safety measures for patients on seizure precautions
      1. Gather seizure history if possible from patient and family or from referral material. Information to be included:
         a. Length of known seizure history
         b. Date of last seizure (type and duration)
         c. Common symptoms experienced
         d. Presence of aura and type
         e. Known precipitating factors
         f. Current medications
         g. Patient and family knowledge
      2. Initiate "seizure precautions"
      3. Initiate safety measures. Place sign, "Seizure Precautions" at patient's bedside and on wheelchair. Tape oral airway to head of bed and back of wheelchair as appropriate.
         Note: This communicates need for seizure precautions to all caregivers and therapists.

Note: These procedures and recommendations were developed by the Department of Nursing at The Rehabilitation Institute at Santa Barbara.

APPENDIX   *(continued)*

    4. Pad side rails of bed with cotton blankets or pads as judged necessary.

    5. Notify therapist if protective helmet is needed for patient with skull defect.

    6. Inform caregivers that electronic thermometer is necessary to take patient's temperature. If glass thermometer must be used, temperature must be taken through rectal or axillary route only.

    7. Obtain suction machine for bedside as judged necessary.
Note: Consider this for patients with difficulty with airway protection or at risk for status epilepticus. *Status epilepticus* is a medical emergency in which the patient is unable to regain consciousness between the seizures, thus increasing the risk of cerebral anoxia or pulmonary aspiration.

  B. Identification and treatment of seizures

    1. At onset of symptoms, stay with patient and call for help. Notify physician. Provide for patient's safety. *Note:* Have crash cart brought to bedside.
Major actions: Protect patient from injury and maintain patient airway.

    2. Turn patient's head to side and flex it slightly to facilitate drainage of oral secretions. Insert oral airway.
Note: Oral airway is preferred and is used primarily if status epilepticus occurs. Never attempt to insert airway during patient seizure or if patient's jaw is clenched.

    3. Place pillow or blanket under patient's head.

    4. If possible, turn patient on his or her side.
Note: If patient is in a wheelchair, tilt chair back, remove belt, and slide chair from underneath patient. If patient has a skull defect, turn him or her to opposite side. Remove harmful objects from reach, or pad surfaces that might injure patient. If patient falls, log roll him or her if possible. If fall occurs, institute spinal precautions until directed otherwise by physician.

    5. Loosen restrictive clothing.

    6. Allow freedom of movement of extremities.

    7. Suction patient as needed.

    8. If patient is receiving nutrition through a tube, stop feeding.

    9. Observe and note pattern of seizure, body parts involved, progression, changes in pupils or gaze, presence of

        incontinence, duration of seizure activity, and respiratory involvement.

10. Monitor vital signs (pulse, respiratory rate, and blood pressure) every 15 minutes.
11. If status epilepticus occurs, direct interventions are to:
    a. Establish and maintain a patient airway.
    b. Provide oxygenation—apply oxygen and contact respiratory therapist.
    c. Prevent cardiovascular collapse.
    d. Prevent injury to the patient.
    e. Control seizure activity with IV medication: Prepare patient for IV insertion (IV medications commonly used include diazepam, phenytoin, and phenobarbital and should be available in the emergency drug box or crash cart; normal saline IV fluid is required when phenytoin is given); and monitor and maintain ventilation, hydration, electrolyte balance, and urine output after the medication is given because medications may precipitate respiratory depression or hypotension.
12. Once seizure has subsided, carefully move patient, take vital signs, and monitor every half hour.
13. Allow patient time to sleep. This is a normal reaction.
14. Observe for presence and duration of postictal symptoms:
    a. Paralysis
    b. Somnolence
    c. Aphasia
    d. Headache
    e. Incontinence
15. Monitor for recurrence of seizure activity.
16. When patient wakes, provide orientation and reassurance.

V. Documentation:

A. Document assessment and seizure history on appropriate medical record(s).
B. Document preventive safety measures to be implemented as seizure precautions.
C. For each incident of seizure document:
   1. Onset of symptoms (time, pattern, and duration)
   2. Patient's activity at the time of onset
   3. General description—loss of consciousness, presence of cyanosis
   4. Pupil or gaze changes
   5. Any injuries

APPENDIX   *(continued)*

    6. Postictal symptoms

    7. Notification of physician

    8. Treatment interventions (i.e., application of airway, O_2, IV insertion—size, site), fluids and medications administered, and patient response.

D. Document patient and family education. Include instructions to patient/family about:

    1. The nature of the seizure disorder.

    2. Signs and symptoms of seizure activity, precautions, actions to take, treatment, medication regime including common side effects of medications.

    3. Common precipitating factors (alcohol, patients withdrawing from alcohol, caffeine, lowered blood sugar, fever, stress, and sudden changes in temperature).

    4. Activity limitations (safety needs, use of machinery, and driving restrictions).

E. Complete "unusual occurrence" form.

VI. General Information:

A. *Seizures* are sudden episodes of varying severity precipitated by abnormal, excessive neuronal discharges within the brain. They are characterized by convulsive movements or other motor activity, sensory phenomena, or behavioral abnormalities. Seizures are the result of excessive release of electrical impulses by a group of neurons in different parts of the brain. Seizures are a symptom, not a disease.

B. Common etiological categories in which seizure activity is a symptom include:

    1. Cerebral injuries

    2. Birth injuries

    3. Infectious diseases

    4. Cerebral circulatory disturbances

    5. Cerebral trauma

    6. Neoplasms of the brain

    7. Biochemical imbalances

    8. Drug or alcohol overdose

    9. Medication-induced electrolyte imbalance

    10. Posttraumatic causes. Seizures may also be idiopathic.

C. Seizures are classified as described in Exhibit 3.1.

EXHIBIT 3.1 Seizure Classifications

I. Partial seizures are seizures that involve or begin in one area of the brain.
 A. Partial seizures with elementary symptomatology (seizures that have relatively uncomplicated symptoms; usually the person remains conscious):
  1. With motor symptoms (symptoms affecting the muscles)
  2. With sensory or somatosensory symptoms (symptoms affecting the senses)
  3. With autonomic symptoms (symptoms affecting the internal organs)
  4. Compounded forms (symptoms of more than one of the above types).
 B. Partial seizures with complex symptomatology (partial seizures with more complicated symptoms, usually with some loss of consciousness):
  1. With impairment of consciousness only
  2. With cognitive symptomatology (symptoms affecting thought)
  3. With effective symptomatology (symptoms affecting mood or emotion)
  4. With psychosensory symptomatology (symptoms affecting sense perception such as illusions or hallucinations)
  5. Compound forms (symptoms of more than one of the above types)
 C. Partial seizures secondarily generalized (seizures that begin as partial seizures and then become generalized).

II. Generalized seizures are seizures that involve both sides of the brain:
 A. Absences (brief lapses of consciousness occurring without warning and unaccompanied by prominent movements, as in petit mal).
 B. Bilateral massive epileptic myoclonus (an involuntary jerking contraction of the major muscles).
 C. Infantile spasms (brief muscle spasms in young children).

continued

EXHIBIT 3.1 *(continued)*

    D. Clonic seizures (seizures consisting of jerking movements of the muscles).

    E. Tonic seizures (seizures in which the muscles are rigid).

    F. Tonic–clonic seizures (seizures that begin with muscle rigidity and progress to jerking muscle movement; commonly known as grand mal seizures).

    G. Atonic seizures (seizures in which there is a loss of muscle tone; the person falls to the ground).

    H. Akinetic seizures (seizures in which there is a loss of muscle movement).

III. Unilateral seizures are seizures involving one hemisphere, or half, of the brain and consequently affect one side of the body.

IV. Unclassified epileptic seizures are seizures that, because of incomplete information, cannot be put into a category.

4

Physical Disabilities after Stroke

The next five chapters deal with the functional consequences of stroke. Stroke typically results in impairment, disability, and handicap. The World Health Organization has developed the following definitions:

Impairment—any loss or abnormality of psychological, physical, or anatomical structure or function. Example: paralysis after stroke (Chapter 4)

Disability—any restriction or lack of an ability to perform an activity in the manner or within the range considered normal for a human being. Example: inability to walk after stroke (Chapters 6, 7, and 8)

Handicap—a disadvantage for a given individual, resulting from an impairment or a disability that limits or prevents the fulfillment of a role that is normal (depending on age, sex, and social and cultural factors) for that individual. Example: loss of job after stroke (Chapter 9)

Although these definitions are used in this text, in clinical practice they can be cumbersome and awkward. More often than not, "dysfunction" or "problem" is used to describe the consequences of disease.

Neuromuscular Impairment

Hemiparesis, partial weakness of one side of the body, or *hemiplegia,* complete paralysis of one side, commonly occur after stroke. Indeed the word *plegia* comes from a Greek word meaning "stroke." If all input to a peripheral muscle is lost, the muscle typically feels soft and lax, known as *flaccidity. Muscle tone*—resistance to passive stretch—is typically decreased early in stroke (*hypotonia*), but may later become increased (*hypertonia*). The change from hypotonia to hypertonia usually is associated with a change from decrease or absence of muscle stretch reflexes (*hyporeflexia*) to brisk or repetitive muscle stretch reflexes (*hyperreflexia*). *Spasticity* is a symptom complex of hypertonia and hyperreflexia frequently associated with spontaneous, repetitive muscle contraction and loss of range of motion (ROM).

In the patient with intact cognitive and language abilities, paralysis is easy to diagnosis. If the patient does not understand the spoken word, gestures or written instructions should be used to attempt to obtain desired motor responses. The patient in coma or with severe cognitive impairment cannot respond as required to requests for movement so a motor examination is difficult to perform. In these individuals, presence of muscle wasting, alteration in reflexes, and degree of tone can be used to gain a rough idea of motor function.

Prevention of reinjury to the recovering extremity is of paramount importance. Intravenous placement or phlebotomy must not be done in the weak arm, especially when sensation is impaired, with rare exception. Skin injury should be promptly attended to with appropriate dressings and debridement. Take care to maintain skin moisture using nondrying soap and an appropriate moisturizing lotion. The patient, family, and staff should be instructed to be judicious, though not overly delicate, in treating the extremities involved. Elbow pads protect the elbows of bony individuals. Lapboards and footplates are useful for protecting the extremities when the patient is using a wheelchair.

The spinal injury stepped paradigm Merritt outlines provides a basis for a rational approach for spasticity control in stroke rehabilitation (Figure 4.1).[1] Prevention of nociception and routine active and passive ROM provide the foundation of care. Tone inhibition begins with proper positioning. The arm of the recumbent patient should be placed in abduction and external rotation as much as possible; unfortunately, frequent repositioning is needed to maintain this posture.

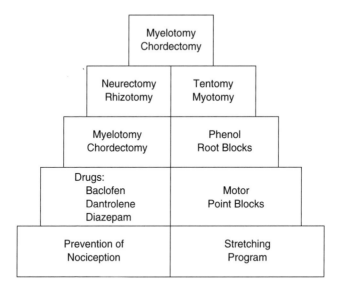

FIGURE 4.1   *Paradigm for spasticity control.*

(From Merritt JL. Management of spasticity in spinal cord injury. Mayo Clin Proc 56:614–622, 1981. Used with permission of the Mayo Clinic, Rochester, MN.)

Lower-extremity weight bearing in transfers and stance or upper-extremity weight bearing through a lapboard decreases hypertonus. Tone-reducing orthotics are available for the arm and leg. Resting hand splints are used, particularly overnight to maintain wrist and hand position. Fully erect posture in stance seems to decrease the tendency for extremity flexion.

Judicious use of medications supplements these physical maneuvers. Dantrolene sodium inhibits the release of calcium ions from the sarcoplasmic reticulum, thus uncoupling excitation-contraction of skeletal muscles. It is generally accepted as the oral medication of first choice in spasticity of cerebral origin. It is not always efficacious, however, as shown by Katrak et al.; and its use may be limited by hepatotoxicity, somnolence, or weakness.[2] Maximal doses (400 mg/day) are often required for best results. Baclofen, a gamma aminobutyric acid (GABA) analog, inhibits monosynaptic and polysynaptic reflexes at spinal and possibly supraspinal levels causing tone inhibition. Although more commonly used in spasticity of spinal origin, baclofen can be used to treat spasticity in stroke, particularly where flexor spasms predominate. Unfortunately oral baclofen often causes unacceptable somnolence. Intrathecal baclofen has been used effectively in children with cerebral spasticity, especially that due to cerebral palsy[3] continuous intrathecal infusion of baclofen for spasticity due to stroke may be available soon. Clonidine, a centrally acting alpha adrenergic agonist used primarily as an antihypertensive agent, also facilitates spasticity control, presumably through reinforcement of descending inhibitory pathways. Its use for stroke patients is not well established. Benzodiazepines, such as diazepam, have played a role in the past, but availability of other agents with fewer side effects and less potential for abuse now limit their use.

Procedural interventions for spasticity control include motor-point blockade, nerve blockade, subarachnoid or paravertebral block, and advanced surgical procedures such as tenotomy, myotomy, cordectomy, or myelotomy. Peripheral blockade is most commonly used in the rehabilitation of the stroke patient. Motor-point blockade provides tone control to a discrete muscle such as the biceps brachii. Nerve blockade can be used to control spasticity in a group of muscles innervated by the same peripheral nerve such as the sciatic. In both situations, electromyography is used to isolate the area to be blocked. Phenol or other substances are then injected into this area to interrupt neuromuscular transmission. Localized botulinum toxin injection is also used in spasticity management.

Electrical stimulation to enhance motor recovery remains controversial. Although there is no question that stimulation results in muscle contraction, there is little evidence to confirm neural recircuiting as a result. Prolonged electrical stimulation to a paretic limb can maintain muscle bulk, but is cumbersome, time-consuming, and sometimes painful. Daily six-hour electrical stimulation to the supraspinatus and posterior deltoid of flaccid stroke patients also receiving conventional physical therapy resulted in significant improvement in arm function, electromyographic activity of the posterior deltoid, shoulder ROM, and subluxation compared to controls who received only physical therapy. Electrical stimulation may prevent glenohumeral stretch, thereby decreasing propensity to subluxation, pain, or upper extremity autonomic dysfunction.[4] Functional electrical stimulation to facilitate gains in self-care and mobility is further discussed in Chapter 6.

Extremity Impairment

Extremity swelling is almost universal in paralysis. Most caregivers think of the worst case scenario when determining the etiology of a swollen extremity. Although shoulder–hand syndrome and deep venous thrombosis (DVT) are potentially devastating, most extremity swelling is due to more benign causes. The majority of swelling is caused by decreased neural control, which in turn affects muscle contraction and blood flow. A paralyzed muscle cannot generate the force necessary to overcome hydrostatic pressure in the soft tissues. Untreated edema can cause pain and delay functional return. Swelling also may be due to reflex sympathetic dystrophy, phlebitis, malpositioning in bed, wheelchair, standing, soft-tissue or bony trauma, or indicative of cardiovascular or renal disease.

Because swelling may be painful, make the skin more prone to injury, and limit functional gains, a rehabilitation program should have aggressive protocols for evaluation and management of edema. Complicated measurement systems using volumetric analysis, while precise, have limited bedside usefulness. The Appendix in this chapter shows a reliable, accurate upper-extremity edema measurement system that is reproducible and easy to perform. Edema can also be evaluated using frequent circumferential arm, forearm, hand, thigh, leg, and foot measurements. Regardless of the system chosen, a high vigilance should be maintained to quickly note new swelling.

Management of benign swelling because of a loss of neural control requires teamwork. As soon as benign swelling is identified, the patient is started on an edema control program and the family is taught to follow through on recommendations. The swollen arm may respond to upper extremity weight bearing, splinting, and elevation. Arm troughs and lapboards can be used in upper-extremity management to facilitate upper-extremity weight bearing; shoulder slings are used only when prolonged standing is necessary. The upper extremity is maintained in distal elevation on the lapboard. Ice dips and slurries cause vasoconstriction and limit edema. Many lower-extremity garments, such as white surgical stockings, do not provide adequate constriction to overcome hydrostatic pressure and direct edema back to the central circulation. Custom or off-the-shelf upper- and lower-extremity garments such as elasticized gloves (Isotoner® by Aris [Sara Lee], New York, NY) or vasuclar stocking (Fast Fit® by Jobst, Charlottesville, NC) with pressure above 20 mm Hg can result in compression. Unfortunately, these may be difficult to don and doff.

Although theoretically useful, lower-extremity elevation generally is not helpful in controlling leg swelling except in the recumbent patient.

Shoulder subluxation deserves special care and attention. The diagnosis is made clinically by noting a palpable gap between the acromion and the humeral head on the affected side that is more apparent than on the unaffected.[5] Although the exact cause of subluxation remains controversial, it is most likely that this phenomenon is due to changes in tone of the supraspinatus muscle that, in turn, alters glenohumeral joint alignment. As supraspinatus tone returns, subluxation often diminishes. Management of shoulder subluxation follows the guidelines discussed above for benign upper-extremity swelling. A sling is useful for ambulatory patients who sublux when upright. The sling should fit well and be easy to don and doff. An overhead sling, a mobile arm support, lapboard, or arm trough can provide additional support while the patient is seated in a wheelchair.

Sensory Impairments

Sensory deficits are common after stroke. The patient may have hemisensory loss described as impairment of light touch, pin prick, temperature, proprioception, kinesthetic, or vibration sense, singularly or in combination. Even with normal strength, the patient with loss-of-joint position in space may evidence severe disability and functional impairment.

Management of sensory loss begins with a patient-focused system for all caregivers. Bed positioning should be done with care so that a neglected extremity is not caught in the bed rails or under the patient. As visual compensation often is important, lapboards should be clear so as not to obstruct the view of the lower extremities. As sensory loss and inattention often go hand in hand, patients should be approached from the affected side and positioned in bed or the wheelchair so that "the action" is on the involved side.

Specific visual deficits are commonly seen after stroke, often in combination with disorders of perception and neglect. The most dramatic may be a gaze preference where the patient's eyes are consistently turned to one side. In severe cases, the gaze may not even be brought to midline (pupils neutral). *Homonymous hemianopsia* is a visual field deficit whereby half the field is cut as a result of stroke. Variations on this field cut include *quadrantanopsias* and other partial losses of vision. *Diplopia,* loss of visual acuity, and tunnel vision are rare in anterior circulation stroke, but *ptosis* and double vision often are seen after brainstem stroke and obscure vision. *Disorders of visual pursuit* prevent smooth saccadic eye movement when following objects in the visual field. Related deficits of visual processing are dealt with in Chapter 8.

Remediation of visual deficits has received limited attention. Optometrists have focused on therapy designed to improve vision through tailored therapeutic exercise.[6] Although there are probably no controlled studies comparing vision therapy with other interventions, anecdotal reports of significant improvement in vision exist. This training is often done with an occupational therapist in the rehabilitation setting. The patient with diplopia or ptosis may choose to use an eyepatch over either eye or may alternate between eyes. Patients often note changes in vision after stroke and ask about new glasses. Given the improvement that so often occurs in sight, it is a good idea to wait at least six months after stroke for new refraction.

References

1. Merritt JL. Management of spasticity in spinal cord injury. Mayo Clin Proc 56:614–622, 1981.

2. Katrak PH, Cole AMD, Poulos CJ, et al. Objective assessment of spasticity, strength, and function with early exhibition of dantrolene sodium after cerebrovascular accident: A randomized double-blind study. Arch Phys Med Rehabil 73:4–9, 1992.

3. Albright AL, Barron WB, Fasick MP, et al. Continuous intrathecal baclofen infusion for spasticity of cerebral origin. JAMA 270: 2475–2477, 1993.

4. Faghri PD, Rodgers MM, Glaser RM, et al. The effects of functional electrical stimulation on shoulder subluxation, arm function recovery, and shoulder pain in hemiplegic patients. Arch Phys Med Rehabil 75:73–79, 1994.

5. Garrison SJ, Rolak LA, Dorado RR, et al. Rehabilitation of the stroke patient. In: Delisa JA (ed), Rehabilitation Medicine: Principles and Practice (pp 565–584). Philadelphia: Lippincott, 1988.

6. Cohen, AH: The efficacy of optometric vision therapy. Am Optom Assoc J 59:95–105, 1988.

APPENDIX

MEASUREMENT SYSTEM FOR EDEMA EVALUATION AND TREATMENT

I. **Policy:**

The Occupational Therapy Department shall provide equipment and assessment tools for the evaluation and treatment of edema in the upper extremities.

II. **Purpose:**

To provide for treatment and management of edema in an upper extremity (UE) by the occupational therapist (OTR) and/or patient, to prevent development of shoulder–hand syndrome, reflex sympathetic dystrophy, brawny edema, and/or permanent joint range-of-movement (ROM) limitations resulting from chronic edema.

III. **Equipment:**

A. Evaluation
1. Cloth tape measure
2. Edema tapes (inches and cm)
3. Edema record
B. Treatment
1. Hand lotion
2. Towels
3. Elevated arm rests
4. Elasticized gloves
5. Bandages, sponges
6. Elastic bandages
7. Crushed ice
8. Large buckets/pans/containers
9. Pumps
10. Small stool
11. Lapboards
12. Two thermometers
13. Hot and cold water

IV. **Procedure:**

A. Edema Evaluation
1. The OTR assesses edema using the cloth measuring tape for the wrist and palmar circumferences, and in the fingers by using the edema tapes. All measurements are recorded

Note: This particular system was developed by the Occupational Therapy Department at The Rehabilitation Institute at Santa Barbara.

	Unaffected Hand	Affected Hand	Affected Hand	Affected Hand	Affected Hand	Affected Hand	Affected Hand	Affected Hand
Date								
Wrist								
Palmar crease								
Thumb prox phalanx								
Index prox phalanx								
Index mid phalanx								
Middle prox phalanx								
Middle mid phalanx								
Ring prox phalanx								
Ring mid phalanx								
Little prox phalanx								
Little mid phalanx								
Total cm								
cm Diff = grade								

Comments:

Patient Name:
Therapist

Key for Grading Edema—Circumferential Scale:
A. Minimal edema—3–7.9 cm; B. Moderate edema—8–12.9 cm; C. Severe edema—13 cm or more

FIGURE 4.2   *Hand Edema Record Sheet developed by the Occupational Therapy Department at The Rehabilitation Institute at Santa Barbara.*

on a "Hand Edema Record Sheet" (Figure 4.2), with date of evaluation.

2. If only one UE is involved, both UEs should be evaluated initially. The noninvolved extremity will be used as a norm for comparison to evaluate extent and progress of edema in the involved extremity.

3. Wrist/palmar measurement: Begin by measuring wrist and palmar crease. Using cloth measuring tape (centimeter side) like the one shown in Figure 4.3, wrap it around the wrist, just distal to the ulnar styloid, to measure circumference. Palmar crease is measured with the tape positioned around the hand, just proximal to the mid phalanx (MP).

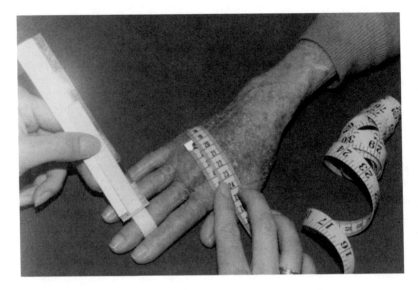

FIGURE 4.3   *Wrist/palmar edema measurement procedure.*

    4. Thumb/finger measurement: Switch to the standard digit circumference edema measuring device (Figure 4.4) for measuring the thumb and four fingers. To measure each digit, slide the cloth loop of the edema measuring device over the digit between MP and proximal interphalangeal joint (PIP), for measuring the proximal phalanx, and between the PIP and distal interphalangeal joint (DIP), for measuring the MP.

B. Treatment

    1. The treatment regime depends on the kind and extent of edema and associated symptoms (i.e., pain, decreased ROM, contractures, amd abnormal sympathetic nervous system responses).

    2. Treatment of the edematous extremity will begin with the least invasive, most conservative techniques. If edema persists, the OTR should utilize other (more aggressive) techniques. The order may be as follows:

        a. Elevation techniques (e.g., lapboard and elevated armrest, pillows in bed, and educating patient and staff to keep arm up on tables, armrests, etc.)

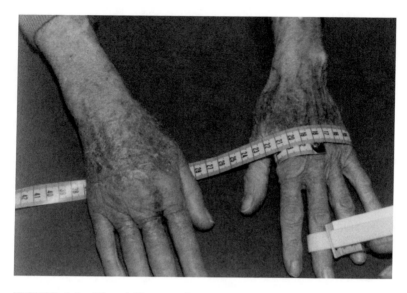

FIGURE 4.4 *Thumb/finger endema measurement procedure.*

> *Note:* In general, slings are not used as a method of ele-
> vation in edema control, because they tend to promote
> flexor synergy and increase spontaneous use of UE,
> which may lead to shoulder–hand syndrome.

   b. Edema massage techniques

   c. Hand pumping and shoulder ROM. Hand pumping
      consists of rapid flexion/extension of fingers (either
      active or passive) up to 20+ times, several times per day.
      This allows the interstitial fluids to flow more freely
      from the hand proximally. Shoulder ROM is done in the
      same manner with more frequent repetitions, as stated
      for hand pumping.

   d. Ice dips

   e. Compression wraps

   f. Jobst® pump

   g. Contrast baths

3. The OTR will leave written (in nursing Kardex) and verbal
   instructions for management of edema with nursing staff
   and patient.

5

Functional Kinesiology

The functional sequelae caused by motor deficits are typically the primary focus of the stroke rehabilitation program. Rehabilitation techniques have been more successful in regaining function in the lower rather than upper extremities. Functional recovery of the hemiplegic arm and hand involves regaining not only motor control, but also proprioception, coordination, and tactile sense. Treatment methods include prevention of complications, as discussed in Chapter 4, neuromuscular facilitation, positioning, therapeutic exercise regimens, functional training, biofeedback, and functional electrical stimulation.

Rehabilitation science has struggled to explain functional gains apart from "natural" neurologic return. Rehabilitation detractors take the view that the stroke patient's neurologic return alone enables functional recovery. Rehabilitation supporters believe therapeutic intervention facilitates natural recovery and achievement of functional gains. We take the latter view, though note that sophisticated scientific evidence of this belief has been hard to come by.

Recovery from central nervous system lesions such as stroke, involves collateral sprouting and neural unmasking.[1] In brief, *collateral sprouting* refers to new growth from intact neurons to a denervated region after some or all of its normal input has been lost.

Unmasking indicates activation of axons and synapses that are present but are not used for the particular function in question—in essence, dormant pathways that are "called up from the reserves" in response to neural injury. Elaborate research is ongoing to define synaptogenesis, neural rearrangement, denervation supersensitivity, neurotransmission, and the role of nerve growth factor(s) in stroke recovery. Observations of stroke patients has led to the following general conclusions:

1. The smaller the lesion, the smaller the deficit (except in the brain stem).

2. Slowly developing lesions create less functional disruption than lesions of the same site and extent sustained suddenly. (For the purpose here, all strokes considered are sudden onset.)

3. Initial deficits after stroke in the young and very old tend to be less marked than those seen in middle-aged people, but deficits in the young often become more pronounced as the neural system matures.[2]

As the patient recovers from stroke, movement returns in characteristic ways. Fugl-Meyer elegantly describe a "method for evaluation of physical performance," specifically identifying the course of motor recovery of flaccid hemiparalysis.[3] He concludes that for most hemiplegic patients the major part of motor recovery takes place within the first months post-stroke, though further improvement may be expected after that period. Fugl-Meyer notes that upper-extremity recovery lags behind lower-extremity function; in his view, the arm will eventually reach the same stage of motor and sensory recovery as that of the leg, a finding we and other authors dispute. He states that the occurrence of joint pain and contracture anticipates poor motor outcome. Although many of Fugl-Meyer's conclusions are dated, the general description of motor and sensory recovery after stroke remains the standard.

Synergy patterns often develop when any flexor muscles of the proximal joints are stretched and distal ipsilateral or contralateral flexion occurs. Similarly, stretch of proximal muscles of extension may result in distal ipsilateral or contralateral extension. As proximal motor recovery occurs, involuntary distal muscles may contract involuntarily, resulting typically in lower-extremity flexion or extension or upper-extremity flexion. Yawning, coughing, or chewing may trigger involuntary movement of the recovering arm or leg.

In 1951 Twitchell wrote what has become the classic description of motor recovery following cerebral stroke.[4] He describes the initial pattern of hemiparesis/plegia, loss of muscle stretch reflexes, and decreased resistance to passive movement. Restoration of motor function begins with return of muscle stretch reflexes, usually within forty-eight hours from stroke onset; increased resistance to passive movement, especially in upper-extremity adductors and flexors and lower-extremity extensors; and clonus. According to Twitchell, motor recovery begins proximally, usually with hip and shoulder flexion, and proceeds distally. Flexion synergies of upper and lower extremities in response to willed effort precedes extensor synergy. As proximal motor control develops, limb spasticity lessens. Upper-limb motor recovery facilitation occurs through proprioceptive reactions, righting reflexes/changes in body positioning, and palmar contactual stimulus. Complete motor recovery results in independence of movement out of synergy, though muscle stretch reflexes may be elevated. Twitchell's description set the stage for the various exercise schools, all of which use some combination of proprioceptive and synergy facilitation or inhibition.

Although some clinicians prefer to inhibit all involuntary reflexes, our view is that some synergy and associative reactions may be encouraged. Synergy patterns can be a double-edged sword. On the one hand, continued flexion may limit distal use and weight bearing; on the other hand, synergy responses may be physically and psychologically useful. In the upper extremity, flexion synergy generally should be inhibited. Lower-extremity extension synergy may facilitate transfers and gait training. It is unclear whether inhibition of synergy truly facilitates isolated motor recovery.

Several neuromuscular facilitation exercise approaches for use in stroke rehabilitation have been developed.[5] Signe *Brunnstrom* utilizes the reflex tensing and synergistic patterns of hemiplegia to improve motor control through central facilitation.[6] She notes that after stroke, limb synergies, primitive postural reflexes, and associated reactions reappear. Upper-extremity flexor synergy consists of scapular retraction and/or elevation, shoulder abduction and external rotation, elbow flexion, forearm supination, and wrist and finger flexion. Upper-extremity extensor synergy consists of scapular protraction, shoulder adduction and internal rotation, elbow extension, forearm pronation, and variable wrist and finger motion. Lower-extremity flexor synergy consists of hip flexion, hip abduction and external rotation, knee flexion, dorsiflexion and inversion of the ankle, and dorsiflexion of the toes. Lower-extremity extensor synergy consists of hip adduction, knee extension, and plantar flexion of the ankle with inversion. Associated reactions are involuntary movement and reflexive increase in tone observed in paralyzed extremities when corresponding body parts on the noninvolved side are resisted during movement. Brunnstrom concludes that these synergies, reflexes, and reactions should be encouraged in the stroke recovery process. Proprioceptive stimuli assist in reinforcing these synergies.

Margaret Rood, on the other hand, used controlled cutaneous sensory stimulation, such as brushing, icing, or tapping, to peripherally facilitate or inhibit motor activity.[7] In *Rood's paradigm,* the normalization of tone is achieved through use of appropriate sensory stimuli. Muscular responses obtained through sensory stimulation are used in development patterns to stimulate supraspinal control of those muscles. Movement obtained is directed toward goal whenever possible. Finally, Rood believes that motor (re)learning occurs through repetition.

D. E. Voss and Margaret Knott introduced *proprioceptive neuromuscular facilitation* (PNF) which advocates the use of neurophysiological mechanisms such as maximum resistance, a quick stretch, and spiral and diagonal patterns.[8] These irradiation patterns place the muscle in a lengthened position, allowing stretching and facilitation. The technique attempts to foster coordination of movement by timing the sequence of muscle contraction within one segment. Maximal resistance promotes irradiation within a pattern. Techniques are applied to enhance movement by position, manual contact, stretch, traction, approximation, and resistance. Demand on the patient is also altered by the use of various tones of voice.

Neurodevelopmental treatment (NDT) is currently the most widely used method. This approach was developed by Karel and Berta Bobath for the treatment of cerebral palsy and only later applied to the management of stroke.[9] Bobath adherents believe that sensation of movement not the movements per se are learned. Abnormal patterns of movement develop because afferent inflow favors contraction of elongated muscles rather than shortened ones. NDT focuses on the inhibition of abnormal tone, postures, and reflex patterns, while facilitating specific automatic motor responses (righting, equilibrium, and protective extension) that will eventually allow the performance of skilled voluntary movements. Emphasis is placed on the three components necessary for skilled movement: normal postural tone, intact reciprocal innervation, and normal patterns of coordination.

All of these approaches are founded in theory. No single approach has been documented as superior for the treatment of stroke, though there is some evidence that PNF is an optimal method in hemiplegia. Most studies looking at efficacy of specific treatment programs have been in the cerebral palsy population, looking at the NDT approach versus traditional exercise. Meta-analysis of these studies demonstrates little difference in outcome. If these data can be extrapolated to stroke, there is likely no one "treatment of choice." The most common clinical practice is to incorporate elements of different methods into the treatment of any individual patient.

One practical method of treatment, the Motor Relearning Programme, incorporates functional training and the identification of key motor tasks such as sitting, standing, standing up, or walking.[10] The therapist analyzes each task, determines the components that cannot be performed, trains the patient in those components and the task, and ensures carryover of this training during daily activities. A type of task-specific physical therapy in acute stroke patients demonstrated more efficacy in improving gait velocity than did conventional neurophysical techniques.

Surgical remediation of functional limitations after stroke has received limited publicity. Despite well-documented improvement in function and physical capacity, surgical intervention generally remains peripheral in most rehabilitation settings. Early reports focused on the surgical remediation of equinovarus, excessive toe curling, planovalgus, excessive hip adduction causing scissoring, and gait stiffness due to rectus femoris tightness.[11] In the upper extremity, surgery may be indicated for flexor tendon, biceps, and triceps lengthening to improve self-care and range of motion.[12] These early studies suffered from lack of long-term follow-up and functional measures. Unfortunately, even a more recent symposium failed to specifically address functional measures of success.[13] To truly confirm the utility of these procedures, more complete studies evaluating surgical, anatomical, and functional gains must be performed.

Motor training should be incorporated into functional activities or else it is wasteful. The aim of rehabilitation is not primarily resumption of movement, but rather resumption of function. The retraining process must increase ease of mobility, self-care, and activities of daily living while developing motor and sensory skill.

References

1. Bach-y-Rita P. Central nervous system lesions. Sprouting and unmasking in rehabilitation. Arch Phys Med Rehabil 62:413–417, 1981.

2. Held JM. Recovery after damage. In: Cohen H (ed), Neuroscience for Rehabilitation (pp 398–405). Philadelphia: Lippincott, 1993.

3. Fugl-Meyer AR, Jääskö L, Leyman I, et al. The post-stroke hemiplegic patient. Scand J Rehabil Med 7:13–31, 1975.

4. Twitchell TE. The restoration of motor function follwoing hemiplegia in man. Brain 74:443–480, 1951.

5. Trombly CA, Scott AD. Occupational Therapy for Physical Dysfunction. Baltimore: Williams & Wilkins, 1977.

6. Brunnstrom S. Movement Therapy in Hemiplegia. New York: Harper & Row, 1970.

7. Rood M. Neurophysiological mechanisms utilized in the treatment of neuromuscular dysfunction. Am J Occup Ther 10:220, 1956.

8. Knott MT, Voss DE. Proprioceptive Neuromuscular Facilitation. New York: Harper & Row, 1968.

9. Bobath B. Adult Hemiplegia Evaluation and Treatment, 3rd ed. Oxford: Butterworh-Heinemann, 1990.

10. Carr JH, Shepherd RB. Chapters 1–3 in A Motor Relearning Programme for Stroke, 2nd ed. (pp 3–42). Oxford: Butterworth–Heinemann, 1982.

11. Waters RL, Perry J, Garland D. Surgical correction of gait abnormalities following stroke. Clin Orthop 131:54–63, 1981.

12. Treanor WJ. Improvement of function in hemiplegia after orthopaedic surgery. Scand J Rehabil Med 13:123–135, 1981.

13. Waters RL, Botte MJ, Jordan C, et al. Rehabilitation of stroke patients—The role of the orthopaedic surgeon. Contemp Orthop 20:311–348, 1990.

APPENDIX

PHYSICAL THERAPY COMMENTARY

Ann E. Veazey, MS, RPT

Although the physical therapist is considered to be one of the team experts in the area of functional mobility training, it is important for each rehabilitation professional to recognize his or her role in providing therapeutic intervention each time the patient is assisted. The vital role of the rehabilitation nurse cannot be underestimated as the one team member who has the opportunity to provide therapeutic intervention on a 24-hour basis. Motor-learning concepts explain what the aims or goals of any therapeutic intervention are:

1. To help the patient move in functional activities with normal patterns of movement;

2. To work toward attaining active automatic movement;

3. To provide repetition so that normal patterns of behavior are learned; and

4. To practice in a variety of contexts so that skills can be transferred to a variety of situations and environments.

Even though it may be "easier" for a patient to use compensatory strategies initially, it is important to teach the patient that the extra effort invested in incorporating the involved extremities into normal functional movements will bring future benefit, allowing for a gain in more functional use of involved extremities and greater ease of movement.

The first step in providing effective treatment/intervention is analyzing which movement components are missing. An understanding of normal movement provides the foundation to accomplish this. Components of normal movement that are missing can be identified by observing the patient move and by handling and moving the patient. These missing components are then facilitated by taking the patient through the movement or functional activity while providing guidance, facilitation, and inhibition to bring about a controlled movement. The treater's input, both manual and verbal, must be monitored consistently for quality and appropriateness to help the patient move normally. The ultimate goal is for the patient to learn new motor patterns that are permanent, automatic, and can transfer to various situations and environments (e.g., bed, car, toilet, dining room chair transfers).

Other concepts to be integrated into daily treatment and intervention include:

1. Providing treatment using meaningful, functional activities (e.g., upright balance while shaving vs. while moving balls or cones).

2. Providing opportunities for weight-bearing and upright function to facilitate midline orientation, and the return of normal tone and control. Upright activities are implemented early during the inpatient stay.

3. Progressively decreasing verbal feedback so that the patient develops his or her own feedback and ability to correct movement errors.

4. Providing opportunities to practice skills in a variety of different situations and environments (e.g., transfer to couch vs. treatment mat).

Gait analysis and training are recognized as a unique area of expertise of the physical therapist. As in any functional mobility activity, the previously discussed motor-learning principles apply to functional ambulation. Orthotic devices may be used initially as "tools" to provide more distal stability in order to focus on developing proximal control and midline orientation. The use of more rigid devices is an area of much discussion among rehabilitation professionals. Although a more rigid orthotic device will inhibit normal motion of the ankle and the body over the base of support, using such a device may initially provide the stability necessary to begin upright activities earlier in the hospital stay and to facilitate practicing more often during the day with various team members.

Treatment should always include transfer and upright activities without devices as well. The physical therapist, orthotist, and physiatrist must continually assess the patient's potential to progress to an orthotic device that allows more normal motion or to using no device at all. The most important concept to keep in mind is that each team member must be invested in providing therapeutic intervention each time the patient is moved or assisted. Applying this concept to daily work with patients, following education and skill development of staff, creates the 24-hour therapeutic environment that ensures the most successful rehabilitation outcomes.

6

Mobility and Self-Care Training

Retraining in mobility and activities of daily living is a primary focus during stroke rehabilitation, from acute care to inpatient rehabilitation to outpatient care and home health services. This chapter discusses general yet practical considerations and approaches in remediating functional deficits caused by strength, sensation, perceptual, visual, and cognitive loss after stroke. Retraining most often incorporates therapeutic exercise and anticipates some return of normal movement; in the severely language or cognitively impaired patient, a purely functional approach is used. Additionally, the treatment approach should involve all members of the rehabilitation team and must be individualized for the patient's medical and neuromuscular status, preferences, habits, social and cultural milieu, economic resources, goals, and discharge plan. Chapter 9 discusses the application of mobility and self-care skills to community living.

Bed Mobility

Bed mobility is an important activity in rehabilitation. Patients need to move adequately in bed so as to prevent pressure sores; protect involved extremities; and position themselves properly for self-care, eating, and other mobility activities. Unfortunately, institutional-based bed mobility training suffers from the unnatural hospital environment. Hospital beds are higher, of different size and firmness, somewhat more mobile, and use different linen. They may also have rails and electric controls that makes mobility easier than in regular beds. Local regulations and fire codes often prohibit use of regular beds in an institutional environment, or modifications such as removal or downsizing of bed wheels that may lower bed height. In this artificial state, the rehabilitationist must endeavor to help patients develop skills that will help them in a home situation.

Independence in bed mobility is often difficult to attain. Cognitive, motor control, motor/sensory processing, and language deficits often adversely affect success. Many patients become frustrated that this seemingly simple activity is difficult to master. Frequent reassurance, creative modification of technique, and group training can enhance chances for success.

For patients who do not recover to a significant extent, compensatory techniques for bed mobility can be used. In order to roll onto the weak side, the patient reaches over the body with the strong arm and pushes off the bed with the strong foot. To roll onto the strong side, the patient grabs the mattress with the hand and pushes against the bed with the strong foot. If necessary, the strong foot hooks the weak foot and pulls it over.

To get up sitting on the side of the bed ("supine to sit or supine to dangle"), the patient slides the stronger foot under the weaker ankle and moves both legs over the same side of the bed on the unaffected side of the body. With the stronger arm the patient grasps the mattress and pushes to sit with elbow and forearm against the bed. The patient then comes to halfsitting, still supporting the body weight on the stronger forearm, scoots the stronger hand posteriorly and pushes to full sit, and uncrosses the legs.

To move from sitting back to lying in bed ("sit to supine"), the patient slides the stronger foot under the weaker ankle while sitting on the side of the bed. With the stronger hand, the patient grabs the mattress and simultaneously lowers the body onto the flexed elbow and swings the legs into the bed. Then the legs are uncrossed and the patient scoots into the desired bed position.

Bear in mind that there are multiple techniques for bed mobility; these compensatory techniques should not be used initially unless it is clear that little recovery is going to occur.

Transfers

The concept of transferring is unfamiliar to most stroke survivors and their families who do not think of moving in and out of a chair or bed as a special activity deserving this cumbersome name. Thus, the rehabilitation provider is placed in the somewhat awkward position of training a patient to perform an admittedly vital activity that in and of itself has little meaning to the patient. Research has shown that many functional successes are built on achievement of transfer skills. Careful explanation of purpose of transfer training can significantly improve task performance and decrease frustration.

Transfer theory has progressed from the dictum "always transfer the patient to her or his strong side" to emphasizing the importance of bilateral transfers that incorporate the hemiparetic side and improve function. Improved theoretical understanding and experience has shown that transfer training can be successful in either direction. Despite awkward names such as "modified Bobath," transfers basically are done with either a squat-pivot or stand-pivot technique. Using a squat-pivot technique, the patient maintains a crouch in coming up from the sitting position; the pivot is performed in this flexed position (Figure 6.1). With stand-pivot technique, the patient comes to a basically full standing position from sitting and may even take small steps during the "pivot" (Figure 6.2).

Experience shows that most problems experienced during transfers include loss of balance when coming to a full stand and difficulty maintaining balance if the patient is unable to control weight bearing on the affected lower extremity. As such, it is best to begin transfer training with significant hip and trunk flexion with anterior pelvic tilt; sometimes rehabilitationists place their upper extremities or chest on the patient's scapulae to prevent "rearing up." Use of an ankle–foot orthosis or air splint may markedly improve transfer skills. While some survivors continue to use particular transfer techniques long after stroke, others continue to improve to the point where transfers once again are seen as part of overall ambulation rather than a distinct activity.

The following transfer activities are part of the scope of training:

- Bed to/from (wheel)chair
- Bed to/from bedside commode or roll-in shower chair
- (wheel)chair to/from commode or shower/bath seat

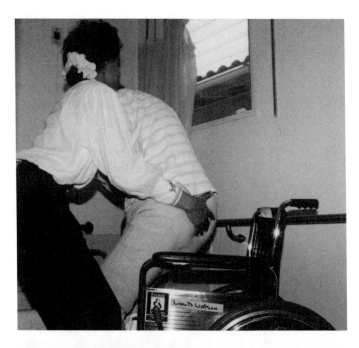

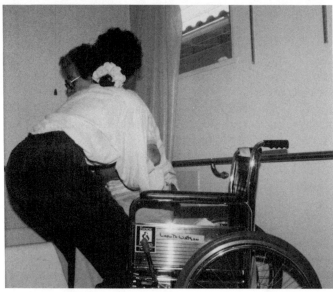

FIGURE 6.1   *Squat-pivot transfer.*

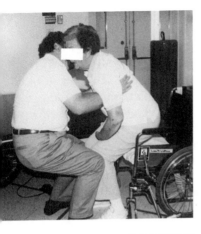
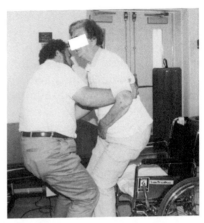
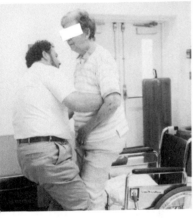
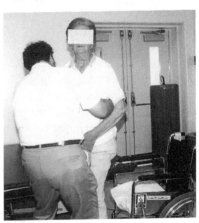

FIGURE 6.2 *Stand-pivot transfer.*

- To/from regular chair
- (wheel)chair or standing to/from car or truck
- (wheel)chair to from floor

There is no such thing as the generic transfer after stroke. Differences in surface heights, friction, and fluctuation in endurance will result in various levels of independence in these transfer activities and perhaps use of different transfer techniques. The rehabilitation team should feel no frustration or inadequacy if the patient's skill level varies throughout the day, provided a consistent approach is used.

Just as patients are often confused when discussing transfers, different staff members may have widely varying views on appropriate transfer technique. At The Rehabilitation Institute at Santa Barbara, no one discipline is in charge of transfers. We try to use the same transfer technique in all situations, but realize that different surface heights and assistant capabilities require modification. Again, caregiver and family training early on should pinpoint problems. Many caregivers worry that transfer assistance will hurt their back; properly performed that should not happen. If this concern dominates discharge planning, a dependent transfer system such as a Hoyer lift or E-Z pivot device may be required. In addition, assistive devices, such as transfer (sliding) boards, have a role in stroke rehabilitation, especially when sitting balance is adequate.

Wheelchair Activities

Stroke survivors have a love–hate relationship with wheelchairs. In the initial phases of rehabilitation, the wheelchair is usually perceived as a temporary device, because most patients expect to ambulate. Later, the wheelchair may be (grudgingly) accepted as a mobility aid. The rehabilitationist must try to understand the patient's view of the wheelchair before wheelchair training is begun.

Wheelchair training is generally divided into three phases: parts, propulsion, and maintenance. Parts training includes familiarization with the various components of the chair and their purpose. During this training, locking the brakes for transfers is emphasized and practiced. Wheelchair propulsion techniques can cause controversy within the rehabilitation team. The classic hemiplegic technique of unilateral arm and leg propulsion serves the majority of stroke patients. Others lack the coordination or simply prefer to use one leg, one arm, both legs, or a combination of all functioning extremities. These later approaches, while often efficacious, may undermine tone-inhibition or neuromuscular strategies. Again, the rehabilitation team should come to a group consensus about the appropriate technique, taking into account the patient's preferences and abilities as well as neurological considerations. Propulsion training and propulsion must occur on a wide variety of smooth, uneven, and inclined surfaces (see Chapter 9). During the maintenance phase, the therapist teaches the stroke survivor and caregiver(s) to survey the brake pads for wear, look for tears and fatigue in the seat and back, and note bent spokes and rough surfaces. It can be helpful for the wheelchair vendor and repairer to meet with the patient at this time.

Wheelchair fitting requires attention to the patient's size, leg length when seated, shoulder and hand status, and planned use of attachments such as the clear lapboard, overhead shoulder sling, balanced forearm orthosis, and/or arm trough.[1] It is particularly important that the patient's feet adequately touch the floor when sitting so that forward propulsion with knee flexion can be accomplished with the unaffected leg. The standard hemi-chair with a 17.75-inch height or ultra-low hemi-chair with 15.5-inch height provides this feature for some patients, but tall adults require taller chairs and short people require shorter chairs—adult chairs with smaller casters or "child's" chairs (Figure 6.3). Obviously, when issuing a wheelchair, the provider also must take the height of the wheelchair cushion into account.

Most stroke patients require brake extensions on the affected side, swingaway leg rests, and pivoting foot rests. Elevating leg rests do not significantly relieve lower-extremity edema despite common use for this indication. Generally, wheelchairs impair good posture because of the sling back and seat. As such, it is important to incorporate firm inserts or replacements such as lumbar rolls, support cushions, and rigid backs. Wheelchair needs may change as the patient progresses; a chair that does not allow significant modification and flexibility should not be procured.

Wheelchair safety is imperative. Chairs with high centers of gravity are more likely to tip than those lower to the ground. Anti-tippers help prevent backward falls. While in the hospital, it is generally a good ideas to use safety belts as supports for wheelchair positioning. Because some may view these as a restraint, it is important to carefully explain their safety function to patients and their families. Patients with marked impulsivity require special attention. For these patients, every activity must be approached cautiously so that recklessness does not cause accidents. These patients often require wheelchair safety belts in the home setting.

Patients with visual neglect and/or field deficit may find wheelchair propulsion challenging. These patients are apt to run into objects on their affected side, resulting in potential injury to themselves or others. Various methods, such as placing a blinking light or brightly colored object in the affected field, have been tried without unequivocal success. It is best to supervise and guide this group closely and endeavor to protect them with full lapboards while allowing wheelchair propulsion without physical restraint.

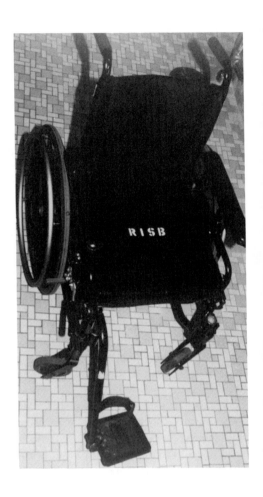

FIGURE 6.3   *Standard hemi-chair.*

Ambulation

Most patients entering stroke rehabilitation want to walk. Fortunately, 70 percent of all stroke survivors regain the ability to ambulate; given the severity of deficit usually seen in rehabilitation inpatients, the percentage of patients treated in a comprehensive program who walk is less.

Esquenazi and Hirai review salient aspects of gait after stroke.[2] Generally, we follow a similar system in restoring ambulation. In the past, rehabilitationists have often described the "hemiplegic gait" as if there is only one type of walking pattern after stroke. Experience shows that stroke survivors present with myriad combinations of motor dyscontrol, spasticity, poor or absent balance reactions, alteration in center of gravity and midline orientation, musculoskeletal change, and strength and sensation loss that result in a decrease in gait quality and speed and potential compromise of safety. Moreover, ambulation at normal speeds after stroke requires a significant increase in energy expenditure; most stroke survivors who walk accommodate for this by walking more slowly. Individualized gait assessment and therapy prescription is imperative in this population.

Normal gait is separated into stance and swing phases. The *stance* phase begins with initial (heel) contact and continues through foot flat, heel off, and toe off. At this point, the *swing* phase begins and subsequently ends with the next initial contact. *Stride* is the period from initial contact to next initial contact of the same foot. Step is the period from a gait event in one foot to the same event in the contralateral foot. During double support, both feet are on the ground; during single support, only one foot contacts the ground. In running there is no period of double support.

After stroke, gait is characterized by one or more of the following: decreased speed, shorter stride, increased swing time, shorter stance phase, decreased weight bearing on the involved side, decreased single support time, and increased stance time on the unaffected side. Foot, ankle, knee, and/or hip movements are significantly altered because of changes in neuromuscular control. Combinations of abnormal toe extension; ankle inversion and plantarflexion; knee flexion and extension; and hip flexion, adduction, and abduction (circumduction) characterize gait after stroke. Toe extension in stance compromises propulsion. *Equinovarus,* the combination of forced ankle plantarflexion with inversion, interferes with stance and swing resulting in initial contact with forefoot or midfoot, poor heel off, and toe drag. Abnormal knee flexion, particularly in stance, produces limb instability. Abnormal knee extension, because of spasticity, plantar flexion contracture, and/or as a compensation for weakness leads to poor contralateral limb advancement, poor weight shifting over the involved limb, and tripping. Inadequate hip flexion in swing, results in toe drag. Over the long haul, these neuromuscular impairments may cause significant joint dysfunction and muscle imbalance.

Weakness itself compromises gait. The patient with weak hip rotators often waddles with a Trendelenburg gait. The patient with weak knee extension finds uneven surface ambulation particularly difficult. The stroke survivor with loss of ankle dorsiflexion may resort to a steppage gait whereby the hip is excessively flexed to provide ankle clearance. Strengthening and bracing can remediate many gait deviations caused by weakness.

Gait training can only begin when patients show enough balance and strength to be reasonably confident in the undertaking. Setting a foundation with strengthening and flexibility exercises bears fruit with the attainment of gait goals. It is crucial to remember that expectations for gait must reflect the patients' desires, medical stability, and discharge plan. Although household ambulation is perfectly adequate for many patients, others must walk in the community to be considered successful.

Assistive devices facilitate safe and efficient gait. It is best to begin gait training at the height-adjustable electrical mat, in the parallel bars, or with a handrail, and progress to front-wheeled walkers, wide- and narrow-base four-prong canes, and single-point canes preferentially. Experience shows that hemiwalkers are not useful in stroke rehabilitation. Standard pick-up walkers, four-wheeled walkers, or walkers with seats rarely benefit the stroke survivor.

Lower-extremity orthotics have proven exceptionally helpful in returning the stroke survivor to ambulation. We rarely use any device other than an ankle–foot orthosis (AFO) because usually patients are able to attain adequate ankle and knee control with this device. Important components of this orthotic include amount of dorsiflexion or plantar flexion and presence of dorsiflexion or plantarflexion stops. Rigid (static) AFOs are manufactured in varying angles at the ankle. An AFO in a few degrees of plantarflexion promotes knee extension (and stability) at initial contact using the principle of ground-reactive force; conversely, plantarflexion may contribute to toe drag during swing and results in unnatural tibial alignment. A rigid AFO set in a few degrees of ankle dorsiflexion promotes knee flexion during initial contact yet improves toe clearance during swing. Articulated AFOs permit some degree of movement within a prescribed angle. Plantarflexion limitation prevents knee extension; dorsiflexion limitation prevents knee flexion.

Prefabricated (off-the-shelf) orthotics can provide acceptable bracing for many stroke survivors (Figure 6.4). These devices can be modified to a minor extent by heating them. Custom orthotics are indicated for hard-to-fit limbs, patients with dynamic edema, and where specialized components or adjustability are required (Figure 6.5). Premade AFOs cost around $300; custom devices range from $600 to over $1,000 (Figure 6.6).

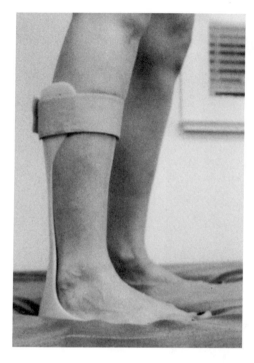

FIGURE 6.4 *Prefabricated ankle–foot orthosis.*

Orthotic needs change as rehabilitation progresses. Many patients initially are served by a static device but later require an articulated or electrically augmented device. AFOs are also indicated to facilitate transfers.

No discussion of lower-extremity orthotics would be complete without a comment on the seeming controversy between plastic and leather/metal devices. Plastic offers lighter weight, total contact, ability to be reshaped and remolded, and improved cosmesis; leather/metal devices offer durability and adjustability. A plastic AFO with dual channel joints offers adjustability with lighter weight. There is no question that each material can be fabricated into an orthotic that serves the patient well. It is important to approach this problem collaboratively and pragmatically using the desire of the treating therapist and the skill and preference of the designated orthotist as the criteria. The rehabilitationist needs to know the expertise of a number of orthotists because insurers are increasingly centralizing orthotic services with preferred providers.

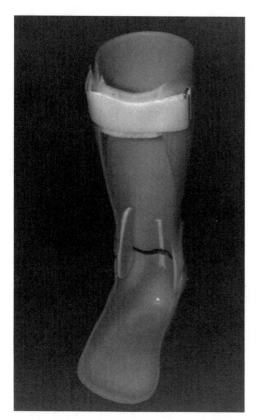

FIGURE 6.5   *Custom, articulated ankle–foot orthosis.*

Biofeedback and electrical stimulation can improve aspects of gait after stroke. Biofeedback has enjoyed a recent resurgence in popularity because of the importance of feedback in learning theory and because of increased interest in "alternative" medicine. With electromyographic feedback, the training focuses on muscle contraction and achievement of strength; electrogoniometric feedback focuses on joint angle, position sense, and improvement in motor control. The earliest electrical stimulation systems to be used as an aid in stroke recovery applied cutaneous stimulation to the peroneal nerve to alleviate foot drop. Subsequent refinements have involved the addition of a heel switch to interrupt the circuit, multiple channels for coordinated stimulation, and partially implantable electrodes with percutaneous connections. To date, no fully implantable, truly functional electrical stimulation system exists.

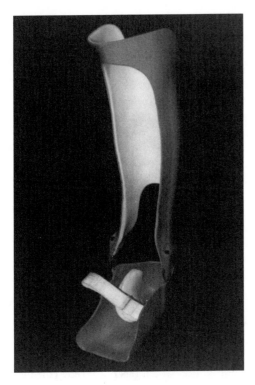

FIGURE 6.6 *Custom derotational floor reaction ankle–foot orthosis.*

Cozean et al. evaluated the efficacy of anterior tibialis and gastrocnemius electrical stimulation and/or electromygraphic biofeedback of anterior tibialis and gastrocnemius in 32 stroke survivors who also received standard rehabilitation physical therapy.[3] They concluded that combined biofeedback and electrical stimulation improved knee and ankle movement during swing and gait velocity more than either modality alone or than standard therapy alone. Morris et al. looked at electrogoniometric biofeedback for genu recurvatum in 26 stroke survivors.[4] They concluded that auditory biofeedback improved subsequent response to later standard physical therapy but did not show statistical significance alone.

Colborne et al. used electrogoniometric feedback of the ankle joint combined with soleus electromyographic feedback in eight long-term stroke survivors in a three-period, crossover design with standard physical therapy as the control.[5] They concluded that the feedback treatments resulted in significant increases in stride length and walking velocity. All these studies suffer from lack of long-term follow-up and correlation outside the laboratory. One of these studies (Cozean) was included in a meta-analysis of eight investigations of electromyographic biofeedback (EMG-BF) characterized by use of randomization and measurement of functional outcome.[6] This analyses concluded that EMG-BF is an effective tool for neuromuscular reeducation in the hemiplegic stroke patient.

While the physical therapist begins the gait training process, other members of the rehabilitation team later contribute their expertise to the attainment of the gait goals. At The Rehabilitation Institute at Santa Barbara, once technique has progressed to a certain point, the physical therapist uses the team conference format and the medical record to enlist the participation of the staff in standing and ambulating the patient. The family and caregivers are involved as early as possible in observing gait training and assisting the patient to walk. Gait training is a long-term process, one that requires seamless service continuity with the home health or outpatient provider. Superlative information flow from the inpatient therapist to other providers facilitates improvement in gait technique after hospital discharge.

For maximal effectiveness, the gains achieved in mobility training must be transferred to the discharge situation. Use of a team communication system and independence log (daily living trials) facilitates keeping track of those activities that the patient has mastered. Through this mechanism, the entire rehabilitation staff and family know not to needlessly help the patient accomplish these tasks. Mobility training in a real-life situation, such as at the shopping mall, grocery store, or at home, best serves the patient's needs. Generally, it is impossible to adequately mimic the community within the hospital walls, so encourage as much activity outside the institution as possible.

Self-Care/Activities of Daily Living

Alteration in strength, sensation, balance, vision, perception, cognition, information processing (agnosia and apraxia), and communication adversely limit the daily activities of the stroke survivor. The rehabilitation team must focus on restoration of appropriate independence in feeding, grooming and hygiene, dressing, undressing, and home management that takes into account the patient's prior patterns and practice. Imposition of a rigid self-care paradigm on an individual patient often leads to frustration and hostility on all sides. Self-care retraining must begin with a thorough inventory of the patient's habits and preferences. From there, critical observation of tasks pinpoints "altered or absent characteristics that impede successful completion."[7] Self-care retraining cannot exist in isolation from mobility and cognitive remediation; program planning should be collaborative.

Feeding is a deceptively complicated activity. Important components that may be impaired after stroke include ability to prepare food for mastication, coordination of upper extremities, visual skills, and ability to self-monitor rate of eating. Issues of dysphagia and nutrition may complicate feeding. Once an assessment of these areas has been completed, retraining may begin in group and individual settings. To assist the patient with cutting and spearing food, rocker knives, plate guards, and friction plates may be used, but be aware that the simultaneous use of rocker knife and fork is dangerous.[8] Many caregivers prefer to cut up food prior to serving it because this saves time; if this definitely is the case, food preparation training should be deferred or avoided.

Many patients do very well using a one-extremity technique of eating or using the affected extremity as an active gross assist; for others with visuoperceptual or judgment problems, this solution is not feasible. Many patients with visual neglect or visual field deficit do not process or see the entire food tray. These patients require auditory and/or visual cueing, placement of plate in the visual field, and plate rotation to completely clear the tray.

Group training in feeding is very beneficial and efficacious but may be difficult with the distractible or impulsive patient or for the person who prefers to eat alone. The hospital tray is not representative of most people's home dining situation. As such, limit use of cartons that require opening, utensils that arrive encased in plastic, and thermal trays; it is preferable to set up tables that resemble a home dining setting. If bibs are needed, all members of the feeding group should use them so that a given patient is not singled out as "sloppy."

Grooming and oral–facial hygiene require safety judgment, depth perception, sequencing skills, upper-extremity dexterity, and coordination. Most grooming training begins at a sink that provides a firm support and stable surface for upper-extremity weight bearing. Wash mitts, suction cups to hold dentures, nail files and other items, electric razors, angled mirrors, dental floss holders, along with myriad other adaptive devices facilitate achievement of independence. Aerosol deodorants, perfumes, and hair sprays are easier to use than pump-dispensed liquids. Environmental simplification through limiting numbers of containers eases self-care. Long-handled grooming aids, such as combs, have not proven effective in long-term use.

Standing training is particularly efficacious at the sink because the patient has visual feedback through the mirror and sees the standing activity as normal and useful. Neuromuscular facilitation should be carried out in sitting or standing during grooming retraining.

Weakness, sensory loss, apraxia and sequencing, language, and cognitive problems converge to make dressing the most difficult task to master after stroke. The clothes the patient wants to wear at home may be significantly different from those required for rehabilitation training; the patient needs to be taught how to don and doff both kinds of apparel. Shirts, robes, dresses, and coats should be loose fitting with the opening down the full length of the front of the garment. Front-opening bras tend to be the easiest to fasten. Dressing sticks make removing clothing from closets easier (Figure 6.7); long-handled shoehorns and stocking aids facilitate dressing. Buttonhooks are useful, but require very secure buttons. Patients with good sitting balance should don and doff lower-extremity clothing while sitting in the (wheel)chair or on edge of bed.

Research has shown that patients often surrender independence in dressing and undressing once home to save time and effort. Even though this happens, it is still important to train patients in this area of self-care; lack of long-term follow-through should not be considered evidence of rehabilitation failure. Malick's very effective description of dressing is shown in this chapter's Appendix.

Stroke patients usually cannot safely stand unsupported in the shower or bathtub. For those with good dynamic standing balance, tub/stall grab bars with friction foot appliques alone provide adequate support. Most patients, though, require some other type of assistive device. Long-handled sponges and hand-held showers with extension hoses have proven very useful for the stroke survivor. A transfer tub bench, with or without a back or additional seat padding, is most appropriate for those who require significant physical assistance and use a squat-pivot or transfer board technique (Figure 6.8). This device fits half inside and half outside the tub. A bath seat with or without a back is appropriate for patients who can step into a shower or over a bathtub ledge. Grab bars inside and outside the tub or shower provide needed additional support (Figure 6.9). For the severely impaired patient who cannot access bathing facilities because of physical or architectural barriers, bed baths provide the best alternative. In general, it is preferable to let a therapist who can treat, or has treated the

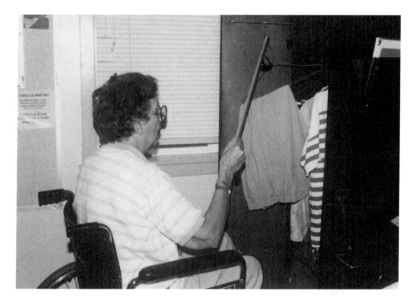

FIGURE 6.7   *Use of a dressing stick to remove clothing from the closet.*

patient in the home, order and install bathroom equipment. Experience shows that therapists who are very familiar with the home situation are best suited to assess the patient's adaptive equipment needs for bathing.

Toileting presents challenges as well. There has been an unfortunate division in rehabilitation between the toileting transfer, clothing management, toilet hygiene technique, and continence, with the nursing service often taking sole responsibility for the later two areas. For the patient, toileting consists of all these components, and requires an awareness of the need to use the bathroom and ability to communicate that need. To that end, all care providers should be encouraged to fully understand and participate in all aspects of the toileting process.

Chapter 3 reviews salient aspects of bowel and bladder care and retraining after stroke. With respect to physical and technical modifications needed after stroke, toilet safety rails, grab bars, and raised toilet seats are effective in increasing independence during toileting. Toilet rails can be easily installed. A three-in-one commode, which provides safety rails and a raised seat, fits into most existing bathrooms and frequently has the added benefit of being covered by insurance (Figure 6.10). Roll-in commodes often have limited usefulness

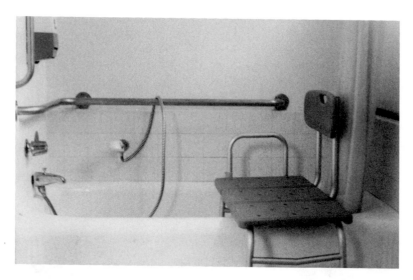

FIGURE 6.8   *Tub transfer bench.*

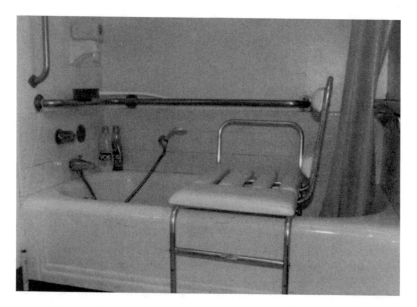

FIGURE 6.9   *Bathroom set up with grab bars, hand-held shower, and extension hose.*

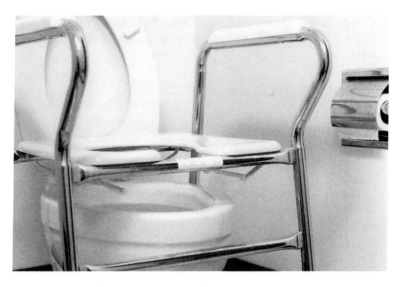

FIGURE 6.10   *Three-in-one commode chair.*

because of poor bathroom access through narrow doors. When bathroom access is limited, the mobility impaired patient usually requires a bedside commode.

Currently, most bathroom equipment is not covered under durable medical equipment (DME) provisions of major insurance policies. Some areas participate in a loan closet program that lends needed equipment to patients; however, many patients must pay out of pocket for these items. Patients often choose to place patio equipment in the bathtub or shower as an inexpensive substitute for bathroom DME. Although this practice is not condoned because of possible safety concerns, it is a frequently utilized approach by stroke survivors.

Conclusion

One size rarely fits all. For best success, the mobility and self-care plan must be individualized with respect to the patient's medical status, habits, and physical disabilities; the rehabilitationist's skills and capabilities; the caregiver's interest, commitment, and desires; and the environment in which the stroke survivor lives or will live. Regardless of the setting—acute-care hospital, inpatient rehabilitation facility, home health care, transitional living center, or outpatient center—the treatment plan must flex to meet the patient's needs.

References

1. Materson RS, Ozer MN. Training in mobility. In: Ozer MN, Materson RS, Caplan LR (eds), Management of Persons with Stroke (pp 367–412). St. Louis: Mosby, 1994.

2. Esquenazi A, Hirai B. Assessment of gait and orthotic prescription. In: Goldberg G (ed), Stroke Rehabilitation. Physical Medicine and Rehabilitation Clinics of North America, vol 2 (pp 473–485). Philadelphia: Saunders, 1991.

3. Cozean CD, Pease WS, Hubbell SL. Biofeedback and functional electrical stimulation in stroke rehabilitation. Arch Phys Med Rehabil 69:401–405, 1988.

4. Morris ME, Matyas TA, Bach TM, et al. Electrogoniometric feedback: Its effect on genu recurvatum in stroke. Arch Phys Med Rehabil 73: 1147–1154, 1992.

5. Colborne GR, Olney SJ, Griffin MP. Feedback of ankle joint angle and soleum electromyography in the rehabilitation of hemiplegic gait. Arch Phys Med Rehabil 74:1100–1106, 1993.

6. Schleenbaker RE, Mainous AG. Electromyographic biofeedback for neuromuscular reeducation in the hemiplegic stroke patient: A meta-analysis. Arch Phys Med Rehabil 74:1301–1304, 1993.

7. Bird C, Mahoney RC. Training in activities of daily living. In: Ozer MN, Materson RS, Caplan LR (eds), Management of Persons with Stroke (pp 346–366). St. Louis: Mosby, 1994.

8. Trombly CA, Scott AD. Occupational Therapy for Physical Dysfunction. Baltimore: Williams & Wilkins, 1977.

9. Malick MH. Activities of daily living and homemaking. In: Hopkins HL, Smith HD (eds), Willard and Spackman's Occupational Therapy, 7th ed. (pp 246–258). Philadelphia: Lippincott, 1988.

APPENDIX

TEACHING PATIENTS DRESSING SKILLS

Shirts, robes, dresses, and coats should be loose fitting with the opening down the full length of the front of the garment.

Method A. Position the unbuttoned garment on lap with the front label of the shirt facing up, the collar closest to the waist, and the armhole for the involved arm centered between legs.

1. Lift involved arm and place it into the armhole.
2. Lean forward so that the involved arm falls completely into the sleeve.
3. Pull the armhole well up above the elbow.
4. Push the remainder of the shirt under involved arm and bring it around the back.
5. Pull shirt onto involved shoulder.
6. Reach back and slip uninvolved arm into the armhole.
7. Adjust the shirt for comfort.
8. Line up the front edges and start buttoning from the bottom, working upward.

Method B. This method tends to be more effective for patients with perceptual deficits.

1. Complete steps 1 to 3 of Method A.
2. Leave the shirt positioned on lap with the front facing upward.
3. Place uninvolved arm into the armhole and push completely into the sleeve.
4. Gather the back of the shirt up to the collar.
5. Lean forward while lifting the shirt up and over head.
6. Pull the shirt down in back and around the chest and adjust for comfort.
7. Line up the front edges and start buttoning the shirt working from the bottom up.
8. Remove shirt from unaffected shoulder and arm before removing from affected arm.

Note: For long-sleeved shirts, cuffs may be buttoned before putting on the shirt. If hands do not fit through the buttoned cuff, sew the buttons on with elastic thread.

APPENDIX   *(continued)*

Lower-extremity underwear and pants usually should be donned while sitting in a wheelchair, chair, or on the edge of bed.

Method A. For the patient getting dressed in wheelchair, chair, or on edge of bed.

1. Cross the involved leg over the uninvolved leg. Balance is best maintained if the involved leg is brought to a point directly in front of the midline of the body.
2. Lean forward and place the underwear over the involved foot and onto the leg. The involved arm may be positioned either on the armrest of the chair or the knee or, if there is increased tone, the involved arm can hang to the side, allowing protraction of the scapula and elbow extension.
3. Uncross the leg.
4. Place the uninvolved foot through the leg hole of the underwear. Pull underwear up over knees.
5. Repeat steps 1 to 4 for donning pants.
6. Before standing, socks and shoes and/or brace should be donned to increase lower-extremity stability.
7. Stand to pull up pants. Place affected arm in pants pocket to prevent garment from dropping to floor. When standing, the patient should have the weight equally on both lower extremities. The therapist should be standing on the hemiplegic side of the patient.
8. Remove pants from uninvolved leg first.

Method B. For the patient who dresses in the bed (for patients who are dependent in transfers, sitting, and standing balance).

1. Put clothing on involved leg first.
2. Bend involved leg at knee and hip using the uninvolved hand. Slip on pant leg, then put uninvolved leg into the other pant leg.
3. Work over the hips either by rolling side to side (roll toward involved side first) or by pulling over the hips with both knees bent. The therapist may need to stabilize the involved leg while the patient pulls the garment over the hips.

Slips and dresses (for women) and undershirt and pullover shirts are donned as follows:

1. Position clothing on lap with neck of garment at the knees and the back of garment on top.

2. Gather the back up into hand until the armhole for the involved arm becomes visible and is located between knees.
3. Lift involved arm up and place it through the armhole. Lean forward, sliding arm between legs into the armhole.
4. Pull the entire sleeve up above elbow.
5. Put the uninvolved arm through sleeve.
6. Lean forward and pull shirt over head.

Socks are donned as follows:
1. Cross involved leg over uninvolved leg.
2. Use the thumb and finger of uninvolved hand to open the sock.
3. Lean forward with the involved arm either hanging at side or bearing weight with the forearm on the involved leg, if the involved arm is unable to assist with this activity.
4. Place the sock over toes and pull it onto foot.

The recommended style for brassieres is a front-opening style which may be easiest to use. Bras can be adapted with hook and loop adhesive to become front-opening. This is the best method for donning the back-opening style:
1. Anchor bra strap with thumb of involved hand, pull opening around to front.
2. Hook bra in front at the waist, remove thumb of involved hand from bra strap, and slip fastener around to the back.
3. Place involved arm through the shoulder strap and then place the uninvolved arm through the other strap. Adjust bra.

Shoes and short leg braces (AFOs) are donned as follows:
1. If patient is dependent in maintaining sitting balance, apply the brace while in bed.
2. Sit in a chair if balance is fair, or on edge of bed if balance is good.
3. Cross the involved leg over the uninvolved leg. Balance is best maintained if the uninvolved leg is brought to a point directly in front of the midline of the body.
4. Make sure shoelaces are loose, then hold shoe underneath the heel. Place it over toes and pull onto heel. (If a short leg brace is attached to the shoe, slip shoe over toes with brace behind the leg.)
5. Uncross legs and place uninvolved hand over the involved hand on top of involved knee and push firmly downward. A long-

APPENDIX   *(continued)*

handled shoehorn in the heel of the shoe may make the process easier.

6. Buckle, tie, or fasten the shoe. Use one-handed shoe tie if vision, perception, and coordination of uninvolved hand is intact.

7. Uncross the legs, and put sock and shoe on uninvolved foot.

(Adapted from Malick, 1988.[9] Used with permission from J.B. Lippincott, Philadelphia.)

7

Swallowing Impairments and Communication after Stroke

Swallowing

Normal swallowing is a complex system of neuromuscular coordination that allows food and liquid to safely pass into the alimentary canal. Alterations in swallowing, including dysphagia and odynophagia, frequently occur after stroke. Although a comprehensive review of the swallowing mechanism is beyond the scope of this book, a basic knowledge of swallowing principles is important for all rehabilitation providers.[1]

There are three phases in swallowing: oral, pharyngeal, and esophageal. The *oral* phase begins when the bolus of food or liquid enters the mouth and continues to the level of the tonsillar pillars. At this point, the pharyngeal phase begins and continues to the beginning of the cervical esophagus. During the oral phase, the bolus is initially masticated and packaged. Once the bolus is prepared, a highly coordinated system propels the bolus posteriorly toward the base of the tongue, closing off the anterior oral cavity in the process, and elevates the soft palate, blocking off the nasopharynx. The *pharyngeal* phase begins with passage of the bolus into the pharynx and consists of posterior movement of the tongue, pharyngeal constriction, laryngeal elevation, epiglottal, false vocal fold and true vocal fold closure, and relaxation of the cricopharyngeal muscle. The pharyngeal constricting wave propels the bolus into the *esophagus* where swallowing is continued by peristalsis.

The incidence of dysphagia after stroke is as high as 50 percent. One third of those will *aspirate*, defined as entrance of material into the airway below the level of the true vocal folds. Of those who aspirate, 40 percent will do so silently, defined as penetration of food below the level of the true vocal cords without cough or other outward sign of difficulty.[2]

Both lower- and upper-motor neuron lesions can result in swallowing dysfunction after stroke. Acute stroke of any type may impair brainstem responses making patients at risk for aspiration. Brainstem stroke may cause direct lower-motor neuron paralysis. Upper-motor neuron impairments may be produced by hemispheric, subcortical, or brainstem infarcts. Moreover, dysphagia can be caused by unilateral or bilateral insults. Patients with brainstem stroke demonstrate a higher incidence of dysphagia than those with other types of strokes. Upper-motor neuron dysfunction may impair the volitional control of chewing, oral transport, and/or pharyngeal swallowing and coordination. As a result, food may enter the pharynx before the initiation of the swallowing reflex. Multiple bilateral strokes causing pseudobulbar palsy may cause spastic dysphagia with decreased speed and delayed initiation of motion. Aspiration can occur in all types of stroke, most often resulting from disturbance in the pharyngeal phase of swallowing related to reduced laryngeal closure, pharyngeal paresis, or reduced pharyngeal peristalsis.

Clinical evaluation of the dysphagic stroke patient begins with a directed history. Of particular concern are complaints of coughing, choking, stridor, and a history of recurrent bronchopulmonary infection. Absence of these symptoms does not indicate safe swallowing. Indeed where there is any concern about dysphagia and alertness, it is prudent to make the patient NPO (nothing by mouth) until additional studies are done. Examination begins with assessment of mental status (especially level of alertness, attention, and concentration), ability to cooperate, language function, memory, visuoperceptual skills, cognitive function, and speech and vocal quality assessment. The muscles of the face, mouth, and neck are examined for weakness, speed of movement, and coordination. Inspection and palpation of the oral cavity serves to rule out dryness, ulcers, growths, atrophy or fasciculation. Gag and pathologic brain stem reflexes should be noted. Direct or indirect laryngoscopy allows care providers to view the more posterior areas of the oropharynx.

Physical examination alone does not fully evaluate laryngeal penetration or aspiration. Swallowing observation supplements data derived from physical examination. At The Rehabilitation Institute at Santa Barbara, the speech-language pathologist (SLP) assesses swallowing at the bedside. She observes rate of eating, management of saliva and secretions, oral clearance, vocal quality, attention, judgment, ability to cough or clear throat, and facility of swallowing. Of particular note is the wet-hoarse quality of the voice after swallowing because this vocal change is found more commonly than other physical findings in dysphagia; unfortunately, it is not detected in all (silent) aspirators.

The videofluoroscopic swallowing study (VSS), also known as a cookie swallow or modified barium swallow, provides additional information that more fully determines swallowing ability and guides management of dysphagia. Specific indications for this procedure include patients with a wet-hoarse voice quality, recurrent bronchopulmonary complications, difficulty managing secretions, and weight loss. The study evaluates oral transport, velopharyngeal closure, laryngeal protection, pooling in the valleculae and pyriform sinuses (Figure 7.1), brimming of material over the area of aryepiglottic folds, retention of food after swallowing, and epiglottic penetration. During the procedure, the patient swallows different consistencies of barium-laced food or fluids that are tracked in anterior–posterior (AP) and lateral projections. The camera should photograph the seated patient from the hard palate to the cervical esophagus (done on lateral view) and the bolus should be followed down the esophagus to the gastroesophageal junction (done on AP view). Thin liquids challenge the impaired pharynx most and usually are given last; this consistency is the most likely to penetrate the airway. The study is terminated if the patient appears unsafe (becomes unable to breathe) on any given consistency (Figure 7.2). Modifications made at the time of VSS include alterations in food volume, method of delivery (cup or spoon), rate of delivery, physical characteristics of the food (temperature or odor), head and neck position, tracheostomy site change, and respiratory maneuvers.[3] The effect of these changes is easily observed and tested immediately; if proven useful, these may be used in subsequent swallowing training.

At most facilities, members of various clinical disciplines are involved in swallowing evaluation and treatment. Of paramount importance is a system of "early warning" for dysphagia and potential

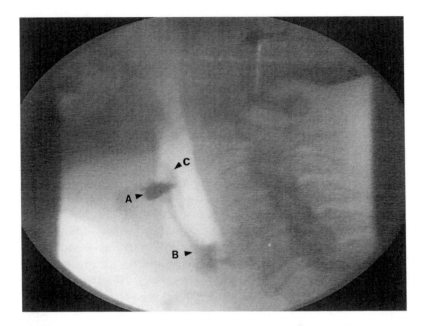

FIGURE 7.1   *VSS showing vallecular pooling (A) and overflow into pyriform sinuses (B). Note outline of epiglottis (C).*

aspiration. Patients with current or previous history of aspiration, esophageal reflux, tracheostomy or feeding tube, chronic obstructive pulmonary disease in conjunction with alcohol abuse, or difficulty handling oral secretions are tagged on admission by any individual treating them as high risk for aspiration. This system is also activated if the initial SLP bedside dysphagia evaluation raises concerns. A protocol of "Aspiration Precautions" is then initiated through which all treaters are informed of potential risk of aspiration and precaution signs are posted at bedside, wheelchair, and activity board. Aspiration precautions consist of:

1. Keeping head of bed elevated at least 30 degrees at all times and 90 degrees for eating or drinking
2. Encouraging frequent coughing and deep breathing, if mouth is clear
3. Supervising feeding and liquids
4. Avoiding use of straws

The need for continued precautions should be reviewed weekly.

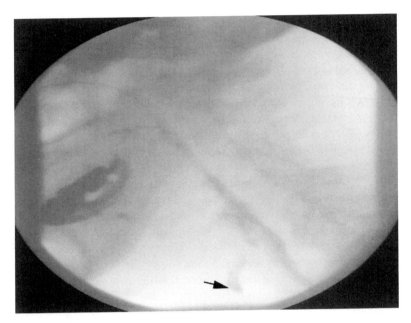

FIGURE 7.2   *VSS demonstrating laryngeal penetration (aspiration).*

Treatment of dysphagia includes oral–motor exercises for the tongue and lips to increase strength, range, velocity and precision, range-of-motion training, and phonation exercise. Drooling of saliva may be decreased by propantheline or glycopyrrolate. If pharyngeal stage function is adequate, loss of food from lip-seal failure, pathologic cervical flexion, or thoracic kyphosis may be compensated by positioning the patient so that the floor of the mouth drains toward the pharynx.

Individual and/or group therapeutic feeding, using chin tuck, double swallow, and other techniques found effective on VSS, are used to treat dysphagia. However, if the food enters the pyriform sinus during pharyngeal swallow delay, the chances that chin tuck will eliminate aspiration are reduced. Faucial arch thermal stimulation has been advocated but has not been shown to definitively restore swallowing capacity. Typically, dysphagia groups occur at breakfast and lunch; these groups can be managed by a speech-language pathologist (see Appendix for more details on the role of SLPs, registered nurse, or properly trained aide. Impulsive and distractible patients often eat, drink, and chew rapidly; retain food in the mouth; overload the pharynx; and fail to appreciate the importance of eating. These patients often need more individualized treatment to force concentration on swallowing retraining.

Patients who aspirate over 10 percent of a test bolus or who have several oral and/or pharyngeal motility problems should have nonoral feeding via nasogastric (NG), gastric, or jejunostomy tubes. Whether a NG tube interferes with swallowing is currently unclear. Nasogastric tubes increase nursing care and may predispose to aspiration, especially if a patient pulls the tube out with the feeding pump on. Also, NG tubes may end up in the lungs rather than the stomach; confirmation of tube location must be done on placement and with subsequent use. If rapid or reasonable progress toward swallowing rehabilitation is unlikely, a gastrostomy for feeding tube placement should be performed within days or weeks rather than months after the diagnosis. The surgical gastrostomy tube is usually easier to change but improvement in design has resulted in less dislodgment of percutaneous endoscopic gastrostomy (PEG) tubes. Protection of the G-tube site with an abdominal binder with a velcro closure is recommended. Patients with large brain stem and significant bilateral hemispheric strokes may remain at high risk of aspiration post-stroke and often require long-term tube feeding. Therapeutic exercises and feeding, as well as repeated swallowing assessment, should continue for these patients.

Speech and Language

Normal speech is accomplished through respiration, phonation, resonation, and articulation. Additionally, effective cognitive functioning is required to produce recognizable speech. Stroke can damage one or more centers vital for the production of intelligible speech. Approximately one third of stroke survivors evidence some defect in speech or language, including aphasia, dysarthria, and apraxias.

Aphasia is an impairment, as a result of brain damage, of the capacity to interpret and formulate multimodal language symbols not attributable to dementia, sensory loss, or motor dysfunction.[4-6] Classification of aphasias can be quite complex; the more common and easily recognized types are listed in Table 7.1.

Assessment and thorough evaluation of aphasia usually falls to an SLP, who evaluates auditory and visual comprehension, verbal language skills, and writing by observation and objective testing. Tests for aphasia, among many others, include the Porch Index of Communicative Abilities, Reading Comprehension Battery for Aphasia, Boston

TABLE 7.1   Classification of Aphasia

Type	Language Characteristics
Nonfluent	
Broca's	Telegraphic, agrammatic expression often associated with apraxia; good comprehension except on more abstract tasks
Transcortical motor	Limited language output; fair naming, intact repetition; fair comprehension
Global	Severe expressive and receptive reduction in language
Mixed transcortical	Severe reduction in expression and reception; repetition intact
Fluent	
Anomia	Word-finding difficulty without other serious linguistic deficits
Conduction	Phonemic paraphrasic errors; good comprehension; fluency in bursts; deficits in repetition of low-probability phrases
Wernicke's	Phonemic and semantic paraphasias; poor comprehension
Transcortical sensory	Fluent neologistic language; poor comprehension; intact repetition

Diagnostic Aphasia Examination, Western Aphasia Battery, and Boston Naming Test. For accurate diagnosis and classification, these examinations should be done in conjunction with cognitive screening. In recent years, there has been a beneficial move away from descriptive classification to a more functional system. The Functional Communication Profile and Communicative Abilities in Daily Living examinations provide more real-life information about communication abilities.[7]

Patients with global aphasia rarely improve significantly; those with Broca's, Wernicke's, and other types can improve. Those who are younger, are in better general health, have less severe aphasia initially, and display good auditory comprehension and preservation of fluent speech improve the most. Techniques used to remediate aphasia include visual action therapy, repetitive auditory stimulation, melodic intonation therapy, verbal language stimulation, hierarchical facilitation of verbal language, and augmentative communication systems such as a communication board and art therapy. Whichever techniques are applied, they must be reinforced by all who are interacting with the patient.

Recently there has been a great deal of interest in the role of the "nondominant" (right) hemisphere in speech and language. The right hemisphere is important for organizing affective behavior. Stroke in this region can result in affective impairments such as denial or levity; cognitive–linguistic impairments in problem solving, memory, and integration; visuoperceptual impairments manifested by altered spatial relationships; hemi-inattention; and dysprosody. *Prosody* is the acoustic signal that communicates the intent of a message through voice pitch, volume, timbre, tempo, intonation, and accent.[8] Normal prosody complements word selection and syntax functions of the left hemisphere. *Dysprosody* is the inability to interpret or apply the nonverbal context of language. The stroke survivor with receptive dysprosody has an impaired ability to recognize the nonverbal aural message being communicated. In expressive dysprosody, the normal inflection and vocal nuance are absent or impaired.

The Rehabilitation Institute of Chicago developed the Communication Problems in Right Hemisphere Dysfunction Evaluation (RICE) to test memory, orientation, perception, pragmatic skills, memory, and integration.[9] This tool is useful in defining deficits in *pragmatic language*—the system of rules delineating language use according to situational contexts. Remediation of right-hemisphere-based language deficits should include memory training and functional problem solving. Experience shows that it is very useful to co-treat these individuals in a group setting that includes both an SLP and an occupational therapist. The group milieu allows support, modeling, identification, and catharsis.

Dysarthria is a common finding after stroke. It is characterized by weak, imprecise, and poorly coordinated speech production with decreased articulation and intelligibility without problems in word retrieval or comprehension. The following Mayo Clinic classification system is widely accepted:

- Flaccid (bulbar)
- Spastic (pseudobulbar)
- Ataxic (cerebellar)
- Hypokinetic (parkinsonian)
- Hyperkinetic (dystonia, chorea)
- Mixed

Dysphonia (as seen in hoarseness) is a related disorder of vocal production, but the problem stems from altered pitch, loudness, quality, and flexibility rather than oral weakness.

A knowledgeable assessment of dysarthria begins with a systemic description of articulation, respiration, resonance, and vocal quality. Intelligible speech is that which is clear, lucid, and understandable. The Assessment of Intelligibility of Dysarthric Speech battery is used to evaluate the effect of dysarthria on the ease and accuracy of understanding speech.[10] The Frenchay Dysarthria Assessment combines an oral–motor examination for strength, coordination, and sensation with a functional speech assessment.[11] Additional testing can include objective measurement of airflow and direct or indirect visualization of the oropharynx, pitch quantifiers, visual biofeedback of speech, or air-pressure transducers, none of which is routinely performed in at most centers.

Treatment of dysarthria is generally beneficial and satisfying. The basic principles are to increase muscle strength, endurance, coordination, and efficiency; improve self-monitoring; provide adaptive strategies; and train caregivers in effective feedback techniques. In general, ataxic dysarthria is treated with steady controlled exhalation, articulatory exercises, rate reduction, and voice exercise. Flaccid dysarthria, as experience shows, is more difficult to treat, may require biofeedback to control airflow, and palatal exercises to improve excursion. If this is not satisfactory, a palatal orthotic can be fabricated to raise the soft palate. Articulatory exercise, respiratory retraining, and resonance and relaxation training are useful in spastic dysarthria. With severe dysarthria, an augmentative communication device may be required. Many different products are available; however, generally, the simpler devices provide more reliability in the long run.

Apraxia, a deficiency in efferent processing, can also complicate speech. Apraxia of speech, also known as *verbal apraxia*—an impairment of voluntary execution of complex speech-motor activities—and *oral apraxia,* a similar impairment specifically involving the oral musculature, are not uncommon. These apraxias can be seen in isolation or with ideomotor, dressing, or other apraxias (see Chapter 8). Inconsistent errors of repetition, omission, and substitution are the hallmark of apraxia of speech. These patients present with overt frustration in communication. Assessment of apraxia requires testing of repetition, oral reading, imitation, and movement of body parts. Dabul's Apraxia Battery for Adults can also be used.[12] Neuromuscular approaches—positioning and facilitation such as melodic intonation—

and phonological approaches to remediate encoding are used in treating apraxia. Experience shows that apraxia is not easily remediable by any specific therapy. Although strategies can be implemented to limit disability caused by apraxia, it appears that improvement stems mostly from neurologic healing. Apraxia can accompany other speech-language disorders, particularly Broca's aphasia (Table 7.2).

The speech- and language-impaired patient needs consistent surveillance and monitoring with routine positive and negative feedback from all rehabilitation providers, family, and friends. Make it a point to educate the family early on in the speech-rehabilitation process and have them participate in therapy often. Interdisciplinary conference time should be used to remind and train staff in the best way to facilitate successful communication.

Rehabilitation for speech and language dysfunction remains controversial. Most improvement in impaired speech occurs in the first six months after stroke, though modest change as late as five years after stroke have been noted. Although most health-care providers generally accept the efficacy of speech therapy in improving functional communication, it is unclear what role spontaneous neurologic recovery may play in restoring speech. Moreover, it is uncertain whether speech therapy facilitates neurologic recovery or only provides adaptive strategies. As such, most SLPs focus both on remediation of specific language impairments and techniques to improve the act of communication.

References

1. Miller RM, Groher ME, Yorkston KM, et al. Speech, language, swallowing, and auditory rehabilitation. In: DeLisa JA (ed), Rehabilitation Medicine: Principles and Practice. Philadelphia: Lippincott, 1988.

2. Teasell RW, Finestone HM, Greene-Finestone L. Dysphagia and nutrition following stroke. In: Teasell RW (ed), Long-term Consequences of Stroke. Physical Medicine and Rehabilitation: State-of-the-Art Reviews, vol 7 (pp 89–100). Philadelphia: Hanley and Belfus, 1993.

3. Shanahan TRK, Logemann JA, Rademaker AW. Chin-down posture effect on aspiration in dysphasic patients. Arch Phys Med Rehabil 74: 736–739, 1993.

TABLE 7.2 Comparison of Aphasia and Apraxia

	Apraxia	*Aphasia*
Definition	A motor–speech disorder	A multimodal language deficit affecting reading, writing, and verbal language
Description	Difficulty sequencing articulatory patterns to say word or move mouth volitionary	Difficulty translating thought into words
Presentation Characterized by	Knows what to say, but can't execute movement 1. Effortful, trial and error, groping articulatory movements, and attempts at self-correction 2. Dysprosody unrelieved by extended periods of normal rhythm, stress, and intonation 3. Articulatory inconsistency on repeated productions of the same utterance. 4. Obvious difficulty initiating utterances	See Figure 7.2
Signs to separate apraxia of speech and conduction aphasia	Difficult to separate because: 1. The severely aphasic patient may not produce sufficient speech to permit identifying the four signs listed here. 2. By definition, apraxia of speech co-exists with Broca's aphasia. 3. Some patients who suffer apraxia of speech have sufficient phrase length and grammatical form to classify them as fluent aphasia.	

(Modified from Rosenbek JC, LaPointe LL, Wertz RT. Aphasia: A Clinical Approach. Boston: College-Hill Press, 1989, pp 87–88.)

4. Morganstein S, Smith MC. Aphasia and right-hemisphere disorders. In: Gordon WA (ed), Stroke Rehabilitation (pp 103–133). Boston: Andover, 1993.

5. Morganstein S, Smith MC. Motor-speech disorders and dysphagia. In: Gordon WA (ed), Stroke Rehabilitation (pp 134–161). Boston: Andover, 1993.

6. Porcelli J. Aphasia assessment and treatment. In: Goldberg G (ed), Stroke Rehabilitation. Physical Medicine and Rehabilitation Clinics of North America, vol 2 (pp 287–300). Philadelphia: Saunders, 1991.

7. Holland AL. Communicative Abilities in Daily Living. Baltimore: University Park Press, 1980.

8. Ross ED. Modulation of affect and nonverbal communication by the right hemisphere. In: Mesulam M (ed), Principles of Behavioral Neurology, 6th ed (pp 239–257). Philadelphia: F. A. Davis, 1985.

9. Burns MS, Halper AS, Muqil S. RIC Evaluation of Communication Problems in Right Hemisphere Dysfunction. Rockville, MD: Aspen Systems Corporation, 1985.

10. Yorkston KM, Beukelman DR. Assessment of Intelligibility in Dysarthric Speech. Tigard, OR: C. C. Publications, Inc., 1981.

11. Endery PM. Frenchay Dysarthria Assessment. San Diego: College Hill Press, 1983.

12. Dabul B. Dabul's Apraxia Battery for Adults. Tigard, OR: C. C. Publications, Inc., 1979.

APPENDIX

SPEECH-LANGUAGE PATHOLOGY COMMENTARY

Joyce Gauvain, MA, CCC-SP

Over the past decade the role of the speech-language pathologist has evolved and expanded into diagnosis, treatment, and management of dysphagia. Treatment involves exercises, thermal application, and learning safe swallowing strategies. Dysphagia can be managed by modifying food and liquid consistencies and position body postures for eating. In cases of dysphagia where aspiration is not considered to be present, the treatment and diet consistencies are often made after a bedside evaluation. If a patient is suspected of aspirating or is showing difficulty with swallowing on a consistent basis, a videofluoroscopic swallowing study needs to be performed. This is the preferred method to determine the exact nature of the swallowing problem and whether aspiration is occurring, and it is available in most community rehabilitation centers. Also, this study allows the therapist to determine what are the safest food and liquid consistencies and best positions for swallowing.

If a patient is aspirating, the timing of the aspiration in relation to the swallow is an important diagnostic, prognostic, and management indictor. Aspiration before the swallow may indicate poor oral control by the patient who loses the leading edge of the bolus over the back of the tongue before a swallow is initiated or the bolus passes into pharynx prior to initiation of swallow reflex (delay in swallow trigger). Tilting chin down for swallow and modifying liquid and food consistencies help in these situations. Remediative therapy would involve oral exercises and/or thermal application.

Aspiration during the swallow can occur because of poor laryngeal closure. Diet consistency modification and laryngeal elevation exercises benefit the patient. If patient is cognitively intact and is good at following directions, the supraglottic swallow may also safeguard the patient from aspiration.

Aspiration after the swallow may occur because of pooling and overflow from the valleculae and/or pyriform sinuses. A double or dry swallow and modifying head position to close off paralyzed side of pharynx may help.

The patient who aspirates need not avoid oral feeding. The cause and timing of aspiration assessed using a VSS study can give vital information for planning appropriate diet consistencies and dysphagia management for the patient to make swallowing as safe as possible.

The primary role of the SLP in treating communication problems is to maximize the overall success of the patient's attempts to communicate. All too often a patient with communication problems will reduce interpersonal contacts or develop counter-productive strategies. It is essential to encourage and support the patient with these difficulties as well as emphasize the most successful modality for him or her by focusing on strengths.

As reviewed in this chapter, dysarthria, apraxia, and aphasia may affect communication after stroke. A patient with dysarthria has intact language skills both receptively and expressively. Speech may be difficult to understand because of muscle weakness and poor breath support.

A patient with verbal/oral apraxia usually will have some degree of co-occurring nonfluent aphasia. Through testing and observation, the SLP will be able to determine the weighting of these two disorders and their effect on communication. A person who is predominately apraxic will have difficulty sequencing sounds but have relatively spared comprehension. A laryngeal-focused apraxia can also occur. This is where the patient has difficulty with motor-planning sequencing to initiate voicing at the level of the vocal folds. A clear, strong cough is heard but the patient cannot volitionally voice for speech production.

A person with aphasia has a language-processing problem. This affects all modalities (i.e., expression, comprehension, reading, writing, and the use of symbolic gestures).

After a right-hemisphere stroke, the pragmatics—the way in which a person uses language in context—may be disrupted. This may be evidenced by tangential irrelevancies in conversation and concentration on specifics instead of a main idea or concept. There may also be a mix–match of verbal expression and motor behavior; a patient may be able to relate a behavior verbally but is not able to execute that behavior appropriately and safely. Such a patient will also lack the insight to assess her or his behavior.

Attention frequently is affected as demonstrated by the inability to carry on a coherent conversation or remember visually and auditorily presented information. Nonverbal aspects of communication may also be affected by stroke, including prosody of speech, facial affect, and eye gaze. Patients with these types of pragmatic deficits may appear disinterested or sad.

Many family members feel a loss or change in the patient's personality. For a stroke survivor with pragmatic deficits, experience shows that it is imperative to improve his or her underlying cognitive deficits as well as the patient's and family member's insight as to what the problems are and how they may impact behavior and outcome.

8

Cognitive, Perceptual, and Sensory-Processing Deficits after Stroke

Cognitive and perceptual sequelae of stroke, including apraxia and agnosia, have a specific impact on physical disability. *Apraxia*—the inability to perform purposefully despite normal coordination, motor function, or sensation—includes constructional, ideomotor, ideational, and dressing types[1] (Table 8.1). As Zoltan states, apraxia may be further categorized by body part affected and class such as transitive, conventional, natural, or nonrepresentative apraxias. Chapter 7 discusses apraxia of speech (verbal apraxia) and oral apraxia.

Agnosia is an inability to identify or perceive a stimulus through sensory means even though its detail can be detected by means of the modality and the person retains relatively normal intellectual capacity. Otherwise stated, agnosia is the inability to interpret or recognize information in one sensory modality when the end organ is intact (Table 8.2). There are many different types of agnosias involving the senses, particularly vision, touch, and hearing.

These information-processing disorders often go unrecognized. It is important to evaluate all stroke patients for color recognition, construction, and visuospatial functioning using a test like the Motor Free Visual Perception Test; visual object recognition of common household products; ability to execute and sequence single- and multi-step motor commands, and skill in object manipulation. Though in the past efforts

TABLE 8.1   Types of Apraxia Common to Brain Injured Patients

Deficit	Clinical Manifestation Resulting Deficit	Treatment
Constructional apraxiagraphic, 2-D or 3-D	Inability to produce designs in 2 or 3 dimensions either on command or spontaneously; patient will be limited in his or her ability to perform purposeful tasks that require use of objects in the environment	Transfer of training approach (i.e., practice copying or constructional tasks); sensory integrative—multisensory (i.e., provide additional proprioceptive and kinesthetic input by having patient draw in a clayboard)
Dressing apraxia	Inability to dress oneself because of disordered body scheme and/or spatial relations; deficit will be manifest by mistakes of orientation of putting clothes on, or neglect	Functional approach with auditory, visual, and/or tactile cueing, and structured repetition; neurodevelopmental techniques (i.e., weight bearing, bilateral tasks, and so on) prior to dressing
Ideomotor apraxia	Inability to imitate gestures or perform purposeful motor tasks although patient fully understands the idea behind the task; patient can carry out habitual tasks automatically	Place tasks on a subcortical level; identify which body parts are affected (i.e., unilateral limb, bilateral limb, total body, and/or buccofacial); provide proprioceptive, kinesthetic, and tactile input before and during the required task
Ideational apraxia	Inability to perform purposeful motor tasks because the patient has lost the understanding of the concept/idea related to the task	Use visualization techniques; use functional approach

(Adapted from Zoltan B. Remediation of visual-perceptual and perceptual-motor deficits. In: Rosenthal M, Griffith ER, Bond MR, et al. (eds), Rehabilitation of the Adult and Child with Traumatic Brain Injury, 2nd ed, Table 24.2, p 354, 1990. Used with permission from F. A. Davis, Philadelphia.)

have been made to pinpoint apraxias and agnosias to certain anatomic regions particularly within the nondominant parietal lobe, it has become clear that any type of cortical stroke (and perhaps even subcor-

TABLE 8.2   Types of Agnosias

Visual Object Agnosias

1. *Apperceptive visual agnosia:* inability to distinguish one shape from another (like a cross from a circle), with ability to see extent of identifying color, movement and direction of movement, line direction and dimension, and light intensity. The patient may gain the information through an auditory, tactile, or olfactory sense.

2. *Associative visual agnosia:* a disturbance in visual recognition with preserved visual perception. The patient can make drawings or copies of objects, but cannot visually identify them.

3. *Tactile agnosia:* inability to recognize objects by handling, despite intact tactile, thermal, kinesthetic, and proprioceptive skills

Apractognosia—loss of perspective

1. *Somatognosia:* lack of awareness of body structure associated with failure to recognize one's parts

2. *Anosognosia:* body neglect to the extent that patient fails to recognize presence or severity of paralysis

3. *Unilateral neglect:* inability to attend to information from one side (usually left) of the body

Auditory agnosia: the inability to differentiate between sounds, despite intact receptive language

Alexia: the inability to ascribe meaning to letters despite intact visual skills; usually not associated with ability to copy letters

Prosopagnosia: the inability to recognize (familiar) faces

Color agnosia: inability to name colors correctly or point to a named color despite intact color perception and memory

Simultanagnosia: inability to simultaneously perceive more than one stimulus item or more than one part of a complex visual pattern

Metamorphopsia: visual distortion of accurately recognized objects (e.g., patient may recognize a chair, but will describe it or its parts as larger or smaller than it actually is)

Finger agnosia: confusion in naming fingers on command

Visual Spatial Agnosias

1. *Topographic disorientation:* despite ability to see and describe a known environment correctly, the patient lacks a sense of familiarity or recognition; inability to understand relationships between places

2. *Position in space:* difficulty in perceived relative position of objects to each other and/or to self

3. Difficulty in *depth perception*

4. *Form perception:* inability to judge variation in form

5. *Figure–ground perception:* inability to separate foreground and background; difficulty in separating extraneous material from matter at hand

tical lesions) can alter sensory processing. For this reason, it is best to look carefully for these problems. In task-specific apraxias, the therapist must look for point of breakdown in a multi-step sequence. Experience shows that diagnosis of sensory processing abnormalities requires vigilant pattern recognition, because apraxias and agnosias generally do not fit into neat categories. Recognition is often a matter of *gestalt*.

After stroke, many patients fail to attend to the involved extremity(ies), presenting with *anosognosia* (neglect of injured body parts). When evaluated, these patients may not identify their arm as their own. Inattention results in failure to adequately protect and position the involved extremity; burns, scrapes, wheelchair accidents, and so on are not uncommon for these patients. More subtly, neglect presents as failure to use a body part that has adequate function for a task that usually would involve that extremity.

Although apraxia and agnosia can be functionally limiting for the stroke survivor, it is important to realize that these same information-processing deficits can impair physical recovery as well. The stroke patient with altered perception may not attend to a weak extremity or might not respond to proprioceptive or other sensory input. As a result, a paralyzed body part may be further injured by a fall, entanglement in wheelchair spokes, or a burn. The patient may "ignore" a swollen hand and not follow through on prescribed self range-of-motion or edema control measures. Disorders of sensory processing impact both physical disabilities and function and should be treated promptly.

It is important to break down functional activities into component parts in order to analyze the underlying mechanisms and subskill of tasks in which deficits are demonstrated. It is imperative to try to focus on the breakdown point of a particular action or task. If gains can be made with specific task components, the patient can often accomplish the entire task or activity under investigation. Treatment, especially of apraxias, should incorporate functional, habitual activities in their appropriate context and setting. Once diagnosed, treatment of apraxias and agnosias focuses on increasing sensory information using alternate sensory pathways such as touch; repetitive functional training; body scheme reorientation using weight bearing, mirrors, or videotape; and performing tasks bilaterally. Typically, a combination of neurodevelopmental, sensory integrative, functional, and transfer-of-training approaches best facilitates recovery.

Remediation of task-specific apraxias is discussed in Chapter 6. Apraxia of gait can be treated with painted horizontal projections attached to straight canes and by marking colored stripes on the floor.[2]

Families and caregivers must be instructed that apraxias and agnosias result from the stroke and are not secondary to willfulness or petulance.

Attention (this discussion refers to overall attention rather than unilateral neglect or hemi-inattention) is a vital skill that enables retention and processing of new information from which memory proceeds. In order of complexity, attention can be measured in terms of ability to concentrate on one topic or object, to shift back and forth from multiple topics or objects, or to simultaneously deal with two or more topics or objects. Initially, it was felt that attention is related to arousal; by implication an "attention center" would be found in the reticular activating system. Laboratory and clinical experience have subsequently demonstrated a broader generalization of attention areas within the brain. Though initially described in right-hemisphere strokes and subarachnoid hemorrhage, attention deficits can be seen in all types of strokes in various anatomic distributions. Attentional skills can be assessed through simple concentration tasks—arithmetic, saying the months of the year forward and backward—and by more subjective measures such as ability to follow a story with or without distraction or tendency for thoughts to wander.

Classic learning theory has separated attention and memory. Memory is divided into three steps: *encoding* (restructuring information into storable form), *storage* (the actual maintenance of stored memories), and *retrieval* (extracting the desired information from storage). Deficits in attention cause difficulty beginning the encoding process whereas memory difficulties may affect all three areas. It is often difficult to formally separate memory processing because the vast majority of objective testing works from retrieval. Additionally, memory is divided into three types: *immediate* (repeating a phone number), *recent* (recalling the events of the day), and *remote* (recalling the name of a childhood friend). Whereas immediate memory is an electrical process that does not require synthesis of new proteins, long-term memory depends on the synthesis of new or increased synthesis of already existing proteins.[3] It has become clear that memory problems, as with apraxias and agnosias, often represent information-processing disorders.

Memory testing can be accomplished in many ways. The Mini-Mental Status Examination can be used as a simple screening test; but, it is insensitive to mild deficits, is influenced by education and age, and emphasizes language. More complicated neuropsychological tests, including the Wechsler Adult Intelligence Battery–Revised, cover memory as part of the comprehensive assessment.[4] The Rivermead Behavioral Memory Test has been found to be particularly useful.[5]

Remediation of memory loss involves cognitive retraining and adaptation. Although repetitious, "drill" work, is useful to increase cognitive capacity. Many rehabilitation centers use log books as memory aids. Therapists, patients, and families are expected to write down thoughts or activities in these books; these entries can be referred to later. This venture is good in theory, but in practice log books are often forgotten or incomplete. Caregivers, therefore, need to be very selective in choosing patients for memory aids. Using the team conference format can be an effective way to remind and cajole members of the rehabilitation team to maintain the log book.

Memory and attention deficits may result in or be associated with disorders of insight, safety, and judgment. *Lack of insight,* the inability to discern the true nature of a situation, may result in patients making false assumptions about their physical capacities and about a particular condition. Patients may then attempt activities far beyond their physical prowess and find themselves in unforeseen territory or even in jeopardy. *Judgment,* the capacity to make sound and reasonable decisions by distinguishing and evaluating data, may also be impaired, resulting in potentially unsafe actions.

For the short term, unsafe patients may require bed or wheelchair restraint; these should be used as little as possible because such devices often increase confusion, agitation, and resistiveness. Infrared bed monitors have not been proven useful in avoiding falls and other adverse consequences of poor safety awareness. Wandering is a particular risk for hospitalized patients who are ambulatory or wheelchair mobile. Vigorous restriction generally increases the desire to flee. Most facilities place a long pole on the back of the wheelchair and a horizontal bar near the top of the doorframes; should the patient attempt to leave a given area, exit is blocked when the pole hits the bar. The treating staff can easily remove patients from the confined area by tilting the wheelchair back about 15 degrees; anti-tipper devices on the chair prevent patients from tipping themselves over. An electronic motion-sensing device prevents egress by emitting a loud noise when specially monitored patients pass near sensory panels. This device's benefits are immediate staff notification and patient behavior modification.

Long-term treatment of safety, judgment, and insight problems focuses on restoration of internal control. Several methods can be used to improve these deficits including behavior modification, role-playing, and didactic problem solving. Family members play a tremendous role here because patients often respond better to reassurances and corrections from them than from the rehabilitation staff. Educating the family and promoting their participation in safety/judgment retraining benefits the stroke survivor and may decrease conflicts between family and staff in this difficult-to-manage area.

The natural history of cognitive-perceptual deficits after stroke has received limited attention. Egelko et al. tracked such deficits in domains of visuospatial perception and reaction time in 58 patients exposed to a standard rehabilitation inpatient program.[6] As expected, right-brain stroke survivors showed more impairment than left-brain stroke patients. They noted improvement in hemispatial neglect from time of initial rehabilitation to follow-up about one year later. Reaction time changed little during this same interval.

Even though progress is often slow and limited in apraxia, task-oriented retraining should be undertaken with these patients. Most stroke survivors (and therapists) find apraxias and agnosias very frustrating. Although some treators prefer to wait until the deficit clears spontaneously, it is best to use early intervention to limit the physical and functional consequences of sensory-processing disorders.

Stroke can cause, contribute to, or co-exist with dementia. Stroke may be a cause of cognitive impairment as with multiple or large infarcts or with infarcts in a strategic location. Stroke may add to cognitive dysfunction by unmasking, modifying, or aggravating underlying impairment. Stroke may also co-exist with dementia with no cause or effect.[4]

References

1. Zoltan B. Remediation of visual-perceptual and perceptual-motor deficits. In: Rosenthal M, Griffith ER, Bond MR, et al. (eds), Rehabilitation of the Adult and Child with Traumatic Brain Injury, 2nd ed (pp 351–365). Philadelphia: F. A. Davis, 1990.

2. Jantra P, Monga TN, Press JM, et al. Management of apraxic gait in a stroke patient. Arch Phys Med Rehabil 73:95–97, 1992.

3. Brinton RD. Learning and memory. In: Cohen H (ed), Neuroscience for Rehabilitation (pp 247–281). Philadelphia: Lippincott, 1993.

4. Erkinjuntii T, Hachinski VC. Dementia post-stroke. In: Teasell RW (ed), Long-term Consequences of Stroke. Physical Medicine and Rehabilitation: State-of-the-Art Reviews, vol 7 (pp 195–212), 1993.

5. Wilson B, Cockburn J, Baddeley A. Rivermead Behavioural Memory Test. London: Thames Valley Test, 1985.

6. Egelko S, Simon D, Riley E, et al. First year after stroke: Tracking cognitive and affective deficits. Arch Phys Med Rehabil 70:297–302, 1989.

APPENDIX

Occupational Therapy Commentary

Sue Ellen Adams, OTR

It is difficult to specifically evaluate apraxia and agnosias secondary to language impairments and overlying cognitive deficits that must be ruled out. With these types of deficits, it is best to rely less on formal testing and more on functional performance for both evaluation and treatment. Creating hypothetical situations is not generally understood.

It is essential to treat apraxia with functional activities in context. Treatment approaches should emphasize physical cues and guiding as opposed to verbal instruction. Often initiation is impaired and guiding facilitates the patient's ability to move on to the next step within a task. This allows for automatic responses to take over to complete a task.

The prognosis for independence with functional activities is different depending on the specific type of apraxia. In motor/ideomotor apraxia the patient does well in familiar surroundings with familiar objects. Past habitual tasks can be engaged in automatically and successfully completed with little or no cueing if the environment is structured appropriately. With ideational apraxia the prognosis is less favorable because of the lack of automatic carryover and the lack of understanding of the concept of the activity. These patients may require constant verbal and physical cues to complete even the simplest functional tasks.

Attentional skills are the foundation of higher levels of cognition. In therapy, we frequently work on the various levels of attentional skills first. However, it is not necessary to adhere strictly to the cognitive hierarchy in treatment which recommends mastering all areas of attention first before moving on to sequencing, categorizing, organization, memory, and problem-solving and executive-functions skill areas. It is possible to focus on one particular level of the cognitive hierarchy, but still provide treatment modalities that address some higher-level areas at an optimum challenge level for the patient.

Whereas treatment for apraxia and agnosia is concentrated in functional activity, treatment for cognitive/perceptual deficits incorporates a variety of modalities including, but not limited to: computer activities, paper-and-pencil activities, self-care, higher-level ADLs, craft projects, and community activities. Treatment for higher-level cognitive dysfunction poses an added challenge because these patients typically function quite well on the ward and in the structured setting of the hospital. Therapy focuses on independent living trials that may involve meal planning and preparation; predriving and behind-the-wheel driving evaluations/training; prevocational activities; and independent use of assistive devices such as log books, calendars, and schedule books.

9

Reintegration after Stroke

Successful rehabilitation of a stroke patient results in community reintegration. The recovery process cannot be considered complete without some degree of participation in the survivor's former world and lifestyle. The degree of disability and handicap seen after stroke is affected by prestroke level of function, medical complications, stroke-related impairments, psychosocial factors, extent of physical recovery, and age. To ensure maximal chance for meaningful participation in the community, reintegration must begin as quickly as feasible.

When discussing post-stroke disability, one must consider the patients' functional status prior to stroke.[1] The elderly, who most commonly have strokes, often evidence loss of community mobility, incontinence, psychosocial loss, and compromise of activities of daily living (ADL) before stroke. One study has shown that 50 percent of stroke survivors achieve complete functional independence four months after the acute event. Of the other half who failed to achieve such independence, 40 percent were disabled for other reasons prior to the onset of their stroke.

In general, survivors with marked physical loss and multiple medical co-morbidities (cardiopulmonary, genitourinary disease, and so forth) access the community less than those with lesser degrees of impairment. Severity of neurological deficits as measured by weakness, cognitive loss, apraxia, and visuoperceptual change correlates with social isolation. Obesity, fractures (often due to falls in the home), and poor cardiopulmonary health compromise participation.[2] Patients and social systems committed to reintegration utilize community services more than those for whom reentry is a lesser priority. Women, those with higher levels of education, and those cared for by a spouse rather than someone else socialize less than their counterparts. Although most stroke survivors fail to achieve previous social levels, most judge their quality of life as good.

Community reintegration requires practice. It is important to take patients on therapeutic outings beginning early in the rehabilitation stay. Initially, the mobility tasks emphasize wheelchair propulsion on various surfaces. As patients progress, ambulation is introduced emphasizing gait-related problem solving in common situations. Community-oriented ADL training emphasizes dining out, accessing financial services (banks, ATMs), general errands (post office), and shopping (groceries, sundries). Sometimes, the techniques learned in the therapy gym do not readily translate to a real-world situation. The community therapist must be prepared to change strategies and should speak with other treators so that the treatment plan can be modified to better meet patients' needs.

Anything can happen on community outings. Patients become hungry and want to eat, or need to use the bathroom. Patients may fall or complain of fatigue and not be able to continue with the activity. Experience shows that community reintegration requires tremendous knowledge and creativity on the part of treators. Every problem that demands immediate attention must be solved safely and quickly to the benefit of patients. The staff attending patients on outings must be able to think on their feet. The entire team benefits when community experiences, successes and failures, are incorporated into the treatment plan.

Many services exist to facilitate reentry after stroke. Referral to community support groups, home health care, community (often geriatric) centers, adult day programs that provide medical and social services, energy assistance programs, errand services, senior planning services, food stamps, grocery delivery, computer database for disability resources, legal services for the elderly and disabled, meals on wheels, respite care, telephone assistance, and van services is useful. The American Heart Association (AHA) and National Stroke Association (NSA) provide valuable educational and referral services for stroke survivors and their families. Generally, community services oriented mostly to stroke survivors prove more helpful than those for the disabled community at large. Santa Barbara is fortunate to have Project Re-entry— a resocialization, client-directed service providing counseling, resource referral, peer support, and leisure activities specifically for stroke survivors and their families. Included in their service is a semester-long training and education course for families and volunteers.

Leisure/Avocation

Active leisure is an important facet of life. Unfortunately, many stroke survivors are not afforded the opportunity to overcome obstacles that limit avocational reentry. The stroke rehabilitation program should offer therapeutic and adaptive leisure reeducation, activities, and referral that provide a diversionary outlet and facilitate functional and neurologic gains. The assessment process should evaluate patients' interests and desires. Although many patients respond positively, others find this focus offputting and inappropriate. For those patients who have difficulty visualizing themselves engaged in hobbies, crafts, and diversionary activities, education using peer support, videotape, and books is imperative.

Many avocational pursuits can easily be adapted for the disabled. Sports—golf, horseback riding, tennis—and table-top games, such as bingo and cards, can be made enjoyable and therapeutic through education and equipment modifications (e.g., cardholders when needed). Large-print and audio books enable resumption of reading. Adaptive art and music activities may allow expression not otherwise available for aphasic patients. Modified gardening using raised beds and adaptive equipment provides diversion and coordination training.[3] In short, there are few activities that are off-limits to stroke survivors; most patients can return to some of their premorbid interests with relatively minor modifications.

Pool activities are therapeutic and diversionary. The buoyancy of the water permits active- and passive-joint movement often not feasible on land. Many patients experience their first success at ambulation in a pool, making the activity particularly gratifying for them and the therapist. Moreover, the pool allows flexibility, strengthening, and aerobic exercise. Patients may enter and leave the pool in a dependent fashion using a Hoyer lift (D. Hoyer & Co., Oshkosh, WI) or, with greater degrees of independence, using steps with a handrail or a ladder.

Cultural Considerations

Most stroke rehabilitation programs adequately address individual and family issues, but often ignore the larger culture from which the patient came and to which the patient is returning. As society becomes more culturally diverse, more and more patients who do not share the Western biomedical view of health and illness participate in the health-care system.[4] Despite use of an interdisciplinary model, North American medical rehabilitation functions within a biomedical paradigm and utilizes the Western worldview of health and disease.[5] Rehabilitation tends to be individually focused, often overlooking the role of the cultural group to which the stroke survivor will return. In a heterogenous society, increasing numbers do not share the same perceptions that inform Western rehabilitation, yet they often conceal their view from providers. As such, providers and patients may find themselves at cross purposes in the rehabilitation setting.

When patient and provider hold differing ideas about health and illness, the ability to provide care may be greatly reduced. In particular, groups differ as to origin of disease. The understandings an individual holds about an illness, called *explanatory models,* illuminate cause, timing, onset, physical processes, natural course, and prognosis of disease. *Personalistic* explanatory models believe illness to be caused by some personal being; *naturalistic* models (like modern biomedicine) explain illness in systemic, impersonal terms. Table 9.1 illustrates differing perceptions of stroke causation. Personalistic systems focus on ultimate cause(s); naturalistic systems focus on immediate cause(s).

Naive realism and stereotyping, two common assumptions, create difficulties in multicultural health-care delivery. *Naive realism,* the view that all people experience the world in basically and same way, and *stereotyping,* the assumption that all members of a group share the same characteristics, limit communication. It is just as ridiculous to believe that all white men will respond in the same way to stroke rehabilitation as it is to believe that all Hispanics, blacks, or other groups respond uniformly.

Components of cultural assessment include evaluation of potential cultural conflicts, appraisal of the patient's health-care beliefs and behaviors, and determination of the meaning of the current medical condition. Efforts should be made to incorporate the patient's beliefs, values, diet, and customs into the care plan. Culturally reliable edu-

TABLE 9.1   Models of Stroke Causation

Cause	Personalistic	Naturalistic
Immediate	—	Cerebral hemorrhage
Underlying	Enmity with neighbor	Hypertension
Ultimate	Moral or spiritual dysfunction	—

cational materials for the patient and family improve understanding and facilitate compliance with the prescribed treatment regimen.

Multicultural and multilingual staff can greatly aid the provision of appropriate care. Unfortunately, cultural diversity has not dominated the employment practices of health-care providers. In 1991, minorities constituted 22% of the U.S. population, but only 8% of practicing physicians, 10% of health administration students, and 14.2% of nursing (RN) school enrollments.[6] Bilingual staff members who only translate words cannot provide truly bicultural services that foster understanding about a patient's health beliefs and practices.

Fortunately, through openness and education, providers can improve the ability to care for those from differing cultural perspectives. The internal case management department often takes the lead in completing a cultural assessment. Careful questioning of and interaction with the patient and family system provide meaningful, accurate information that then can be disseminated to the rehabilitation team. Outside medical anthropology and public health consultants can offer useful, straightforward tips for the rehabilitation system.

Vocational Issues

Between 3% and 84% of stroke survivors return to work. The reasons for this broad numeric spread include disparity in the definition of work, demographic heterogeneity of groups compared, patient selection, differences in intensity of restorative services received, and cultural factors.[7] Vocational intervention can be important for all survivors of stroke, particularly the 25% of stroke patients who are between 45 and 65 years of age. The decision to return to work may be delayed for several months as neurologic and functional recovery proceeds.

Negative predictive factors for return to work include aphasia, poorer nonverbal reasoning skills, lower Barthel index scores, longer rehabilitation stays, nonwhite race, and alcohol use.[1,5] Psychological and social variables, such as degree of helplessness, loss or role, shame, and lack of family support, may limit vocational reentry. Side of hemiplegia, gender, and age do not consistently predict return to work. Younger patients with less residual disability are more likely to return to work than older patients. Similarly, management-level employees are more likely to return to work than laborers.

Many services facilitate job reentry after stroke. These programs may include functional, cognitive, and physical training; vocational assessment; and job coaching. An active program of supportive employment training—intensive time-limited training, compensatory strategies, extended assessment, and retention tactics—seem to assist stroke survivors' return to employment.[5] It has been found that a supportive employer is vital if the stroke survivor is to return to the workforce. If a stroke occurred during the course of employment or during activities of employment, the worker's compensation system may be the primary provider of vocational rehabilitation services; for many other situations, state employment programs are the only source for vocational reentry training.

Sexuality

Many stroke survivors want to resume sexual activity but often fail to do so because of fear of stroke recurrence, embarrassment, depression, and loss of confidence. Unfortunately, the sex lives and practices of many older patients have often been limited by these premorbid health factors; stroke creates further constraints, usually to the point of sexual activity cessation.[8] From a medical perspective, diabetes, particularly with peripheral nervous system impairment, heart disease, hypertension, and medications are much more restrictive in limiting sexual performance than stroke per se or side of lesion. Serum level of sex hormones do not change after stroke.

Nonetheless, male and female stroke survivors report a decline in libido, foreplay activity and intercourse frequency, erectile and orgasmic dysfunction, sexual satisfaction, vaginal lubrication, feelings of unattractiveness, and a decrease in caressive expressions.[9,10]

Alterations in sexual drive and performance seem due to psychodynamic, social, and general medical problems including fatigue, bowel and bladder dysfunction, depression, anxiety, altered body image, self-esteem, and changes in role and spousal relationships.[11] Post-stroke sexual and relationship problems, such as rejection by the spouse, may reflect premorbid relationship problems more than the direct effect of a stroke and serve to legitimize the subsequent maladaptive patterns.[8] Men report more dissatisfaction with sex after stroke than women, perhaps because women are more culturally conditioned to resign themselves to the changes described here.

At The Rehabilitation Institute at Santa Barbara, the psychology department takes the lead in discussing sexual issues with the stroke survivor. A general introduction to sexuality after stroke is provided in the education materials the patient receives on admission. The psychologist later queries the patient as to whether there are additional questions. The topic is also discussed by the nursing staff with the patient prior to therapeutic home passes. Should the patient or family have questions, they are addressed in a forthright, nonjudgmental fashion. The lines of communication must be kept open in the outpatient arena because the majority of sexual activity takes place after hospital discharge. Ongoing education, reassurance, humor, and encouragement (remembering the caveat that, despite rare case reports to the contrary, there is no evidence of an increased incidence of stroke after orgasm) help the patient and partner meet their goals.

As with other aspects of adaptive leisure, lifestyle modification for sexual expression need not be cumbersome or expensive. Verbal and visual education sets the foundation for successful resumption of sexual activity. Attempts should be made to broaden "sex" to "sexuality" thereby adding foreplay, caressing, and intimacy to coitus. Because of balance difficulties and weakness, many male stroke survivors cannot use missionary (man on top) or rear-entry positions easily. However, side entry or man on bottom positions are often very successful. Men who have difficulty achieving and/or maintaining erections may benefit from medications, including papaverine and erectile assistive devices. These devices use a hand- or electric-powered (often preferred if an upper extremity is weak) pump or thick condom-like sac that fits snugly over the penis. When the device is activated forming a vacuum, the penis is engorged and erection ensues. The erection is maintained with ring or tubing constriction. These devices should be used with care and partner supervision if the patient has cognitive or sensory deficits.

Other therapeutic modifications include liberal use of water-based lubricant (particularly for patients with limited fluid intake) or estrogen cream, use of techniques for anxiety control, and efforts to improve communication and assertiveness skills. It is often helpful to plan sexual activity following bladder and bowel emptying. For the patient who is impulsive or easily diverted, every effort should be made to minimize distraction. Compensatory strategies for deficits in visual acuity, perception, mobility, sensation, and memory, using guiding, visual cueing, repetition, and familiar gestures have proven useful.

References

1. Delaney GA, Potter PJ. Disability post-stroke. In: Teasell RW (ed), Long-term Consequences of Stroke. Physical Medicine and Rehabilitation: State-of-the-Art Reviews, vol 7 (pp 27–42). Philadelphia: Hanley & Belfus, 1993.

2. Teasell RW. Long-term Consequences of Stroke. Physical Medicine and Rehabilitation: State-of-the-Art Reviews, vol 7, 1993.

3. Yeomans K. The Able Gardener. Pownal, VT: Storey Communications, Inc., 1992.

4. Barker JC, Clark MM. Cross-cultural medicine a decade later. West J Med 157, 1992.

5. Hoeman SP. Cultural assessment in rehabilitation nursing. Pract Nurs Clin North Am 24(1):277–289, 1989.

6. Sabatino F. Culture shock: Are U.S. hospitals ready? Hospitals (May 20), 1993.

7. Black-Schaeffer RM, Osberg JS. Return to work after stroke: Development of a predictive model. Arch Phys Med Rehabil 71:285–290, 1990.

8. Freda M, Rubinsky H. Sexual function in the stroke survivor. In: Goldberg G (ed), Stroke Rehabilitation. Phys Med Rehabil Clin North Am 2:643–658, 1991.

9. Boldrini P, Basaglia N, Calanca MC. Sexual changes in hemiparetic patients. Arch Phys Med Rehabil 72:202-207, 1991.

10. Monga TN. Sexuality post-stroke. In: Teasell RW (ed), Long-term Consequences of Stroke. Physical Medicine and Rehabilitation: State-of-the-Art Reviews, vol 7 (pp 225–236), 1993.

11. Williams SE, Freer CA. Aphasia: Its effect on marital relationships. Arch Phys Med Rehabil 67:25–52, 1986.

Other Resources

American Heart Association
7320 Greenville Ave.
Dallas, TX 75231
   Stroke: A Guide for the Family
   Up and Around: A Booklet to Aid the Stroke Patient in
                Activities of Daily Living

National Stroke Association
300 E. Hampton Ave., Suite 240
Englewood, CO 80110-2622
303/762-9922
   The Road Ahead: A Stroke Recovery Guide
   Be Stroke Smart

APPENDIX

RECREATION THERAPY COMMENTARY

Kathryn H. Richmond, MS, RTR, CTRS

The majority of individuals who suffer a stroke today will survive as a result of modern rehabilitation techniques and advanced medical expertise. With increased survival rates, strokes have become the leading cause of long-term disability in the United States.[1] To reduce the effects of disability, rehabilitation historically has focused on tasks relating to physical functioning, thus improving basic daily-living skills. The importance of incorporating knowledge of the patient's lifestyle, adjustment, and psychological needs, however, often has been overlooked in some therapy programs. Fear, poor self-image, lack of confidence, motivation, or a myriad of other reasons may preclude the successful application of even basic skills learned in the hospital to the home environment such as bathing, dressing, eating, and mobility.

Reintegration Training

To maximize an individual's successful reintegration into home and community life following a stroke, a comprehensive treatment approach is recommended, incorporating physical, cognitive, social, and psychological components. One treatment method, *reintegration training,* uses an integrative approach that views adjustment arising out of the interaction between the person and his or her social and physical environment. Reintegration training is a transitional rehabilitation approach that includes both the restoration of physical function through a medical restorative model, and reeducation through adaptation of social and living-skill competencies.[2]

The continuum of rehabilitation care a stroke survivor experiences begins with meeting a team of professionals who evaluate the individual's physical, cognitive, psychological, and medical status. One of the team members responsible for facilitating the reintegration process is the recreation therapist. To develop a treatment plan that is pertinent and has long-term carryover, the recreation therapist completes an assessment with the patient and/or significant other. Information includes the patient's prior leisure interests, lifestyle changes as a result of age and/or disability, community involvement, social and family support, and prior motivation for leisure and social involvement. The treatment plan is developed based on assessment information from all team members. Needs are then prioritized based on the patient's goals, the team-identified rehabilitation goals, projected length of stay, resources, and discharge plans.

Therapy may incorporate recreation activities—games, sports, crafts, or music—to improve fine- or gross-motor skills, endurance, memory, and/or social interaction skills. Adaptation of past leisure interests and exploration of new leisure interests takes a more prominent role in the treatment plan as the patient begins to realize the scope of specific impairments. During inpatient rehabilitation, the recreation therapist may suggest a new way of doing something that is first rejected and, months later, finally tried. Examples include:

A 60-year-old business executive who was forced to retire after his stroke as a result of impaired cognitive skills. A year after discharge he called the recreation therapist, saying he had been close to suicide. Loss of status, relationships, and too much time on his hands to think negatively contributed to his downward spiral. Fortunately, he remembered information about a program where he could learn to play golf with only one hand. He was finally ready to try a new way of living and soon began to develop a more positive outlook on all aspects of his life.

A 72-year-old woman who had had many destructive lifestyle habits before her stroke, including overeating, smoking, and lack of exercise. During her rehabilitation program, she learned new leisure skills that helped her maintain her health. She was never a swimmer, but wanted to learn a form of exercise she could do with a flaccid arm and weak leg. She learned to swim and was referred to a community program where she swims three times a week. One day a week she attends a stroke activity group and offers peer support for other people in the rehabilitation program.

Once they return home, most stroke patients have an abundance of leisure time, either temporarily or permanently. Teaching the patient and family how to manage leisure time in a constructive way that will sustain and improve physical and emotional well-being is important to reduce the chance of a significant decline in function after discharge. Without some ongoing efforts on the part of the patients, the benefits of the rehabilitation program can quickly be nullified by problems of adjusting to the residual deficits from a stroke.

Teaching home leisure skills is just one area of reintegration training. Early in the patient's rehabilitation program, reorientation to the world outside the hospital is initiated. Integration of all therapy skills is then practiced in the community.

Community Reintegration Training

The recreation therapist works with the patient, family, and team members to facilitate the carryover of skills learned in the clinic to the community. Such skills include transfers, mobility, dressing, eating, speech, problem solving, and bowel and bladder management. The recreation therapist may teach the patient "street smarts" because what works in the accessible hospital bathroom may not work in a restaurant bathroom. Helping the person realize that he or she can solve problems and manage needs safely in the community may prevent an individual or family from becoming homebound unnecessarily.

Community reintegration training is designed to provide sequential challenges, education, and skill development and accomplishment. Patients are encouraged to take control of their lives, making choices and decisions. Most importantt, patients and family members experience life outside of the hospital environment and begin to address social and emotional issues of disability as well as lifestyle changes. CRT is an opportunity for the family to come together and try new skills with the supervision and guidance of a therapist. As it progresses, this training leads to passes for the family to go out for a drive or to visit the patient's home.

Family Training

The effects of a stroke are felt by the whole family; therefore, teaching every member what the stroke survivor can do is important. Training family members increases their confidence and understanding of how to assist, as well as how to avoid enabling the person to "learn to be helpless."[3] Wheelchair management on curbs and in restaurants, theaters, and stores is one area of training. Information pertaining to the health benefits of maintaining physical and social outlets is shared, while recreation and community resources for future use are provided.

Summary

The comprehensive approach of reintegration training focuses a team effort on what is necessary for patient and family to resume as independent a lifestyle as possible. The combination of therapy techniques that result in the amelioration of function and the adaptation to the environment is the key to reducing the potentially negative and costly effects of long-term disability.

References

1. National Institute of Neurological and Communicative Disorders and Stroke. Ther Recreation J (April), 1993.
2. Callahan M. The Effects of a Community Reintegration Program on Patient Functional Outcomes. Paper presented at Annual Therapeutic Recreation Conference, Anaheim, CA, 1988.
3. Seligman MEP. Helplessness: On depression, development and death. San Francisco: Freeman Company, 1975.

Suggested Reading

Berryman D, Trader B. Benefits of Therapeutic Recreation in Physical Rehabilitation: A Consensus View. A paper from conference proceedings sponsored by United States Department of Education and Temple University's Therapeutic Recreation Program, 1991.

Armstrong M, Lauzen S. Community Integration Program Manual, 2nd ed. Seattle: Harborview Medical Center, 1994.

MacNeil R, Pringnitz T. The role of therapeutic recreation in stroke rehabilitation. Ther Recreation J (April):153, 1993.

Niemi ML. Quality of life four years after stroke. Stroke 19(9):1101–1107, 1988.

Bullock CC, Howe CZ. A model therapeutic recreation program for the reintegration of persons with disabilities into the community. Ther Recreation J 25(1):7–17, 1991.

Resources

Stroke activity centers are available in many communities. Contact the local Rehabilitation Center, City Recreation Department, or American Heart Association to locate the closest program. For information on developing a stroke resocialization program, a few model programs in California include:

- The Long Beach Stroke Activity Center
  2800 Studebaker
  El Dorado Community Center
  Long Beach, CA 90815

- Palm Springs Stroke Activity Center
  P.O. Box 355
  Palm Springs, CA 92263
  619/323-7676

- City of Santa Maria Recreation Department Stroke Support
  419 South McClelland
  Santa Maria, CA 93454
  805/925-0951

- Project Re-entry, A Stroke Resocialization Program
  c/o Lorraine McNiece
  3903 Laguna Blanca Drive
  Santa Barbara, CA 93110

10

Psychological and Social Consequences of Stroke

As a direct or indirect result of stroke, the patient and social system may experience any one of a number of psychological and social sequelae. Although these consequences may be trivial, more often than not they markedly increase disability and dependence. Prevention through education and prompt recognition and treatment should be part of any stroke rehabilitation service.

Table 10.1 lists common psychological disturbances seen in stroke patients. *Denial,* a protective emotional mechanism frequently implemented to avoid depression or other psychopathology, is usually present throughout initial inpatient rehabilitation.[1] Most patients entering stroke rehabilitation hope to return to normal; this hope is often reinforced by spontaneous improvement in paralysis. Attempts to confront denial generally prove nonproductive and undermine staff credibility. Moreover, some patients never acknowledge or demonstrate great distress or grief after stroke. The rehabilitation staff should not presume the pain of physical loss and stroke disability or force a patient through a prescribed grief paradigm.

TABLE 10.1   Psychological Disturbances Seen in Stroke Patients

- Denial
- Anxiety
- Depressive disorders
  - Adjustment disorder with depressed mood
  - Dysthymia
  - Major depression
- Catastrophization
- Avoidance
- Indifference
- Undue cheerfulness/sadness and other disturbances in mood
- Emotionalism
- Shame
- Anger
- Dependence

In addition, patients who suffer strokes often experience some or all of the following social changes:

- Social isolation
- Decrease in community involvement
- Economic strain
- Disruption of family life
- Loss of role (at home and/or work)
- Dependency
- Decrease in satisfaction with life in general

Nonetheless, many stroke survivors experience some type of affect response. Depression is seen in 20% to 63% of stroke patients; of those, half are clinically depressed and the other half evidence some type of depressive disorder such as dysthymia.[2-4] Premorbid personality, degree of physical loss, amount of family/community support, loss of self-esteem, guilt, viewing stroke as punishment, and intellectual deterioration contribute to *reactive depression*—a response to loss and uncontrollable events. Yet not all depression is reactive; it is wrong to assume that all post-stroke depression will fade rapidly or without intervention.

Much work has been done to correlate depression with strokes in certain cerebral anatomic distribution. Robinson and colleagues argue that patients with left-hemisphere brain injury were significantly more depressed than patients with right-hemisphere or brainstem infarcts.[5] Other researchers' experience shows that location of brain injury influences psychological reaction to a degree; however, little definitive evidence exists that specific brain location solely determines emotional problems.[6] Right-hemisphere lesions may result in denial, indifference reactions, emotional lability, and euphoria more than left-hemispheric lesions that produce more anxiety and depression. Frontal injuries are more commonly associated with depression and euphoria. Pseudobulbar states are associated with emotional lability. Subcortical and brainstem injuries less commonly lead to direct psychological consequences, though depression has been associated with basal ganglia stroke. In the long term, depression is not related to anatomic localization of infarct. Neurochemical studies have argued for diverse causalities for early and late post-stroke depression. Specifically, catecholamines dysfunction with neurotransmitter asymmetry may be particularly important.

Demographic factors have been related to post-stroke depression. Younger patients were found to have a greater degree of depression than the older ones, perhaps because stroke drastically interrupted the young patients lives and was more expected in the old. Yet there is evidence that depression rates in elderly stroke patients exceed what would be expected based on normal aging alone.[3p549] There does not appear to be a strong association between gender and ethnicity and post-stroke depression.

Recognition of post-stroke depression is difficult. This chapter's authors concur with other reports that post-stroke depression is often underdiagnosed and treated, both in inpatient and outpatient rehabilitation settings. Many of the standard tools for assessing depression have limited usefulness for the post-stroke patient. Vegetative signs, such as disturbance in sleep, appetite, and libido, are present in many stroke patients for a variety of reasons and are too nonspecific to be used to diagnose post-stroke depression. Self-reporting inventories—the Beck Depression Inventory, Hamilton Rating Scale for Depression, and Zung Self-Rating Depression scale—subsume intact cognitive functioning. DSM-IV criteria (Table 10.2) rely partially on behavioral observation and may be the most useful assessment tool. Unfortunately, three of the nine criteria require some verbal response, somewhat undermining the reliability of this test. The dexamethasone depression test does not accurately identify post-stroke depression. Use of a combination of DSM-IV testing and psychological interview in the initial evaluation of potentially depressed patients is recommended.

TABLE 10.2   DSM-IV Diagnostic Criteria for a Major Depression Episode

Note: Criterion A below defines *Major Depressive Syndrome.*

A. At least five of the following symptoms have been present during the same two-week period and represent a change from previous functioning; at least one of the symptoms is either (1) depressed mood, or (2) loss of interest or pleasure. (Do not include symptoms that are clearly due to a physical condition, mood-incongruent delusions or hallucinations, incoherence, or marked loosening of associations.)

  1. Depressed mood (or can be irritable mood in children and adolescents) most of the day, nearly every day, as indicated either by subjective account or observation by others

  2. Markedly diminished interest or pleasure in all, or almost all, activities most of the day, nearly every day, as indicated either by subjective account or observation by others of apathy most of the time

  3. Significant weight loss or weight gain when not dieting (e.g., more than 5 percent of body weight in a month), or decrease or increase in appetite nearly every day (in children, consider failure to make expected weight gains)

  4. Insomnia or hypersomnia nearly every day

  5. Pyschomotor agitation or retardation nearly every day, as observed by others, not merely subjective feelings of restlessness or being slowed down

  6. Fatique or loss of energy nearly every day

  7. Feelings of worthlessness or excessive or inappropriate guilt (which may be delusional) nearly every day (not merely self-reproach or guilt about being sick)

  8. Diminished ability to think or concentrate, or indecisiveness, nearly every day, either by subjective account or as observed by others

  9. Recurrent thoughts of death (not just fear of dying); recurrent suicidal ideation without a specific plan, or a suicide attempt or a specific plan for committing suicide

B. (1) It cannot be established that an organic factor initiated and maintained the disturbance, and (2) the disturbance is not a normal reaction to the death of a loved one (Uncomplicated Bereavement).

  Note: Morbid preoccupation with worthlessness, suicidal ideation, marked functional impairment or psychomotor retardation of prolonged duration suggest bereavement complicated by major depression.

C. At no time during the disturbance have there been delusions or hallucinations for as long as two weeks in the absence of prominent mood symptoms (i.e., before the mood symptoms developed or after they have remitted).

D. Not superimposed on Schizophrenia, Schizophreniform Disorder, Delusional Disorder, or Psychotic Disorder NOS (not otherwise specified).

From *Diagnostic and Statistical Manual of Mental Disorders,* 4th ed. Washington, DC: American Psychiatric Association, 1987. Used with permission.

Treatment of depression is imperative. Depression impedes functional gains just as a lack of functional progress may precipitate depression. Moreover, mood disturbances, feelings of hopelessness and helplessness, and other signs may wear on the patient and deserve intervention. Suicide has been reported in stroke survivors.[7] As mentioned before, depression can be present for many months to years after stroke. The rehabilitation program must provide comprehensive, long-term services to deal with this devastating problem. Fortunately, psychological counseling and medication management are very effective in treating post-stroke depression.

Experience at The Rehabilitation Institute at Santa Barbara shows that combining individual and group psychotherapeutic methods with medication management is most helpful in treating post-stroke depression. Milieu therapy, reminiscence, cognitive therapy to alter interpretation of life events, and behavioral therapy to remind patients of positive life events can be used. The ability of the inpatient psychologist to make a great deal of progress in treatment is limited by shortened acute rehabilitation stays of less than one month. For this reason, an outpatient case manager needs to be involved with discharge planning and outpatient orientation should begin with a session with a marriage, family, and child counselor who can continue to provide treatment and identify new psychological and social issues.

Antidepressants and other medications are often useful in post-stroke depression. Most research in this area has focused on the heterocyclic medications (amitriptyline, nortriptyline, trazodone, others) which have proven useful in relieving depression and improving activities of daily living performance. Unfortunately, there use is limited by anticholinergic side effects of sleepiness, urinary retention, constipation, and dry mouth. Additionally, heterocyclic medications can compromise cardiac rhythm, particularly in the patient with cardiac ischemia and coronary artery disease.[8] It is safe to assume that the vast majority of patients with cerebrovascular disease also have some cardiovascular disease; therefroe, it is advisable to avoid heterocyclic medications when treating post-stroke depression. If they are used, prior to beginning heterocyclic therapy, obtaining an electrocardiogram is recommended.

Selective serotonin reuptake inhibitors (SSRI)—fluoxetine, sertraline, and paroxetine, others—offer an improved safety profile compared to heterocyclics, but have not been specifically tested in stroke patients with depression. Some institutions use these antidepressants preferentially in initial therapy. As a general rule, they are well tolerated and effective. Side effects include anorexia, hyperarousal, and insomnia; additionally, patients often experience a persistent tremor, particularly with fluoxetine.

Other types of medications have proven useful in post-stroke depression. Methylphenidate, an amphetamine derivative, improves attention and arousal. Its quick onset is particularly impressive—when patients are started on this medication, they show improvement in a few days. Generally, it is best to begin treatment at 5 mg two times per day (breakfast and lunch); the highest dose recommended for use with the depressed stroke patient is 10 mg bid. Experience to date shows no cardiac side effects with this medication. Although clinicians do not fully understand the mechanism of action of methylphenidate in post-stroke depression, its effect on arousal improves functional performance and indirectly improves mood and affect.

Emotionalism, defined as emotional lability and weakly yielding to emotion, is present up to one year after stroke in up to 21 percent of patients. Most of those affected cry easily, precipitated by sad or sentimental situations, or by discussion of emotionalism.[6] It is found especially in patients with temporal or left-frontal lesions. The patients affected lose the ability to suppress an emotional response at low levels of stimulation; they often find the resultant crying or undue cheerfulness socially disabling. Treatment includes education of patient, family, and friends as to the nature of the problem, reminding them that the emotionalism is not always inappropriate. It is usually beneficial to stop the conversation at hand or divert attention when emotionalism becomes problematic.

Anxiety and anger are present in 32 percent of stroke patients, usually because of uncertainty about recovery, present affairs, family members, dying, and having another stroke.[7] Anxiety is seen more commonly with cortical strokes. Constant reassurance and tangible feedback of gains made in rehabilitation diminishes anxiety. Benzodiazepines and sedatives are reserved for the highly refractory situation because of their cognitive side effects and deleterious effect on ability to participate in the rehabilitation program. A relatively new medication, the anxiolytic buspirone, has not proven useful with post-stroke anxiety.

Catastrophization involves extremely disruptive emotional outbursts with physical and/or verbal abuse directed toward staff and family. This extreme anxiety reaction occurs rarely, usually in response to physical or cognitive challenge or in those with marked aphasia. The best treatment is to remove the patient from the threatening situation. For patients susceptible to catastrophization, easy and hard tasks should be alternated in therapy and each session should end with a treatment success. Threats of punishment or retaliation aggravate the situation and are contraindicated.

After stroke, social problems include economic strain (46%), social isolation (53%), decreased community involvement (43%), disruption of family function (52%), poor motivation, dependency, and loss of control.[3,9] Social isolation initially results from physical disability (hemiplegia, incontinence) but often continues even when physical problems cease. Mobility, self-care, communication, and cognitive deficits often combine with feelings of inadequate worth and value to limit socialization. Social isolation is more severe in women and in those with higher educational achievement.

Isolation may be heightened by inability to drive. North American lifestyles, with rare exceptions, require frequent use of private vehicles to engage in social activities. Driving represents independence and youth and is a highly valued right by most adults. After stroke, the rehabilitation team may direct the survivor not to drive because of concerns about safety, judgment, insight, and problem solving, as well as deficits in mobility, visual acuity, perception, and balance. Although many patients and families accept this recommendation, the survivor often feels betrayed when told not to drive. State laws vary regarding the rehabilitation provider's responsibility to the Department of Motor Vehicles. In California, the rehabilitationist and attending physician must notify the state of the patient's stroke, in effect voiding the driver's license. The Driver's Safety Office then arranges a behind-the-wheel test to reinstate driving privileges. Until the patient can resume driving, he or she remains dependent on his or her spouse, family, and friends for private transportation. Although public and private accessible transportation is available in most communities, many stroke survivors find it inconvenient and insulting and consequently use it very little.

Stroke takes direct and indirect economic tolls. Home assistance through a home-care agency can cost up to $11.00/hour; through a home health agency, it can cost up to $17.00/hour. Many patients buy long-term care insurance policies only to find that they only cover institutional services; the cost of "unskilled" care provided in the home often comes from family coffers. Most families are unprepared to meet these financial obligations, so they hire live-in attendants and/or do the majority of the work themselves. Many older adults continue to work part-time after formal retirement. A stroke often deprives them of this income source and/or forces the spouse/caregiver to retire.

Stroke is a family matter. Effective family functioning is characterized by mutual concern, good communication skills, trust, balance of power and influence, tempered with love and good humor. The family that functions at such a high level often can effectively deal with the needs of the stroke survivor and facilitate adherence to the stroke rehabilitation program. On the other hand, the dysfunctional family usually does not have the resources to meet the challenge of caring for a disabled stroke survivor in the home. More often than not stroke disrupts family patterns. Successful rehabilitation provides the family with the skills to physically care for the patient and the capacity to creatively cope with this unexpected turn of events.

Family functioning can be assessed through a variety of methods.[10,11] Self-reporting questionnaires that can screen level of family health include the Family Environment Scale. Interview measures, such as the Standardized Clinical Family Interview, involve clinical sessions and offer the advantage of direct observation of family patterns. Evans et al. used the Family Assessment Device, which tests prestroke family interaction, to predict stroke rehabilitation outcome.[12] They found that measurable family factors, such as affective responsiveness and affect control, proved useful in predicting posthospitalization adjustment. Unfortunately, none of these methods is routinely available or feasible in the majority of rehabilitation settings because of staff resource and financial constraints. As such, rehabilitation providers are left to make their best judgment about family patterns by observing conversations. Often, the assumptions made while observing these interactions are wrong or incomplete. The rehabilitationist then plans treatment with an inaccurate view of the family's skills and expectations. For example, a family's uncertainty and emotional distress may result in overinvolvement or coalescence; the therapist mistakenly assumes this family is completely committed and dedicated to life-long caregiving at home.

Poor family support tends to result in increased depression and poor compliance with prescribed post-rehabilitation regimens. Poor functioning can lead to caregiver illness (insomnia, anxiety, "stress") and "burnout" which in turn decreases the resources available to the patient. In severe situations, neglect or abuse may be the result of family collapse.

Conversely, good family support decreases the emotional and physical deterioration of stroke patients and maintains the functional gains of rehabilitation. Good support eases the role change required by the needs of the stroke survivor. Patients with strong family support enjoy more gratifying interpersonal relationships and socialization.[13]

Education is necessary but not sufficient to facilitate successful family caregiving.[14] The rehabilitation program must provide families and caregivers with reliable, useful information on stroke, disability, medical issues, community resources, and psychological and social consequences after stroke. At inpatient facilities, it is important to encourage spousal attendance at a weekly support and educational group designed to acquaint them with the issues they will face. As mentioned before, at The Rehabilitation Institute at Santa Barbara, the outpatient program begins with a psychological and social assessment of patient and spouse in the hopes of pinpointing areas of dysfunction early in the recovery process. An outpatient caregiver's group meets weekly for ongoing support, companionship, and education. Spouses and caregivers with acute needs are treated individually by the psychology staff. Unfortunately, most home health agencies do not offer such a comprehensive program.

Spousal and family counseling seems to facilitate positive changes in family functioning and provides additional benefits in behavioral control and affective involvement.[12] These gains were maintained at one year after inpatient stroke rehabilitation discharge. Counseling has not been shown to significantly decrease subjective burden of care.

The spouse/caregiver requires specialized intervention to maintain optimal performance. Unfortunately, the incidence of depression in spouses of stroke patients is about 2.5 to 3.5 times that of controls.[13] Factors that lead to depression include the assumption of additional responsibilities, the shattering of the "golden years" illusion, financial burden, decreased personal time, and loss of usual companionship and social interactions outside of the home. As a result, marital tension and discord can grow. Survivors with loss of insight, problem solving, and judgment have particular difficulty interacting with their spouses, while the burden on caregivers is associated more with instability in family support than with patient behavioral problems.[14]

Patient and family systems may adjust to stroke through anxiety, denial, acceptance, and assimilation. As mentioned earlier, many stroke survivors go through a grieving process that includes acceptance of the reality of the loss; experiencing the pain of the loss; adjusting to an environment where the lost abilities are obvious; and reinvesting energy in new, feasible activities and social roles. A number of factors contribute to post-stroke behavior and mood, including prestroke behavior, psychological reaction to stroke disability, neurobehavioral deficits, and family supports. Individuals who believe they can control or influence the events of the experience, are committed to the activities of their life, and anticipate change as an exciting challenge adjust more effectively after stroke.

Åström et al. studied quality of life over three years in 50 long-term survivors of stroke.[15] They measured life satisfaction defined by social network, functional ability, leisure-time activities, experience of ill health, and major depression. Compared to the elderly at large, these stroke survivors had lower life satisfaction and functional status. Contacts with family were maintained whereas interactions with friends were dropped, a finding corroborated in clinical practice at The Rehabilitation Institute. Function and neurologic status changed little after the first three months of follow-up; conversely psychological status changed over the first year after stroke. If good life satisfaction was attained during the first year after stroke, it tended to be maintained; poor life satisfaction at one year remained over the entire study period.

To maximize the chances of a satisfying life for stroke survivors and their families, liberal use of community services within the entire first year after stroke should be encouraged. If the challenges of resuming a meaningful life are not met, patients may respond with maladaptive behaviors. Implementation of diverse coping options can maximize restoration of physical and psychosocial function.[16]

Geriatric Concerns

No book on stroke rehabilitation would be complete without a discussion of the specific needs of older adults. With aging, the incidence and prevalence of chronic and multiple diseases increases. Because of scientific advances and aging of the North American population, geriatrics has become a medical specialty. Moreover, it is common for older adults to face unique challenges when confronted with any disability that requires specialized intervention. In the rehabilitation environment, *geriatrics* focuses on elderly who become disabled and the disabled who become elderly.

The growth of the aged population carries special significance because of its implications for disability and its impact on those who provide rehabilitative services. In general, the aged show increased susceptibility to and disability from acute illnesses and injuries. Most studies agree that older adults tend to be more impaired in mobility, physical activities, and daily-living skills than younger adults.

Many false assumptions are made regarding older adults; in fact, only a minority of them become dependent, alienated from their families and support systems, or institutionalized. Ageism—the inaccurate stereotypes made about the elderly and their role in society—contributes to the negative perception of older adults.[17] Common misperceptions include the following:

- Most elderly wish to be cared for by their children.
- Depression is a natural consequence of aging.
- Many illnesses are a natural consequence of aging and do not warrant medical assessment or intervention.
- Most older adults are well-off financially.
- It is inappropriate to discuss end-of-life issues with the elderly or to provide intensive rehabilitation services to older patients who choose to forego aggressive or resuscitative medical care.

Normal aging may produce myriad physiologic changes, including immune system dysfunction and decline in end-organ function. With specific regard to stroke, aging has limited impact on the neurologic and musculoskeletal systems. Loss of short-term memory; loss of speed of motor activities (with slowing in the rate of central information processing); and impairment in stature, proprioception, and gait come with normal aging.[18] Many aspects of learning and memory, including immediate memory and retrieval from long-term storage, remain relatively intact during normal aging. Age-related impairments involving episodic loss of short-term memory have been consistently documented, most likely related to slowing of central processing. It is clear that older adults are capable of new learning, but at a somewhat slower rate. Muscle strength, number of motor units, overall muscle mass, and muscle fiber size decrease with age. Biochemical alteration of cartilage with reduced ability to cushion, ulceration of cartilage, and subsequent exposure of subchondral bone is seen commonly. "Degenerative" joint disease is ubiquitous in older adults; however, many are only mildly symptomatic. All told, these losses often result in functional deficits.

References

1. Swartaman L, Teasell RW. Psychological consequences of stroke. In: Teasell RW (ed), Long-term Consequences of Stroke. Physical Medicine and Rehabilitation: State-of-the-Art Reviews, vol 7 (pp 179–193). Philadelphia: Hanley and Belfus, 1993.

2. Malec JF, Richardson JW, Sinaki M, et al. Types of affective response to stroke. Arch Physical Medicine and Rehabilitation 71:279–284, 1990.

3. Berk SN, Schall RR. Psychosocial factors in stroke rehabilitation. In: Goldberg G (ed), Stroke Rehabilitation. Physical Medicine and Rehabilitation Clinics of North America, vol 2 (pp 547–562), 1991.

4. Price TR. Affective disorders after stroke. Stroke 21(suppl II):12–13, 1990.

5. Robinson RG, Price TR. Post-stroke depressive disorders: A follow-up study of 13 patients. Stroke 13:635–640, 1982.

6. House A, Dennis M, Molyneux A, et al. Emotionalism after stroke. BMJ 298:991–994, 1989.

7. Garden FH, Garrison SJ, Jain A. Assessing suicide risk in stroke patients. Arch Phys Med Rehabil 71:1003–1005, 1990.

8. Glassman AH, Roose SP, Bigger JT. The safety of tricyclic antidepressants in cardiac patients. JAMA 269:2673–2675, 1993.

9. Churchill C. Social problems post stroke. In: Teasell RW (ed), Long-term Consequences of Stroke. Physical Medicine and Rehabilitation: State-of-the-Art Reviews, vol 7 (pp 213–223), 1993.

10. Evans RL, Hendricks RD, Haselkorn JK, et al. The family's role in stroke rehabilitation: A review of the literature. Am J Phys Med Rehabil 71:135–139, 1992.

11. Bishop DS, Evans RL. Family functioning assessment techniques in stroke. Stroke 21(suppl II):II-50–II-51, 1990.

12. Evans RL, Bishop DS, Matlock A. Prestroke family interaction as a predictor of stroke outcome. Arch Phys Med Rehabil 68:508-512, 1987.

13. Teraoka J, Burgard R. Family support and stroke rehabilitation. West J Med 157:665–666, 1992.

14. Evans RL, Bishop RS. Psychosocial outcomes in stroke survivors. Stroke 21(suppl II):II-48–II-49, 1990.

15. Åström M, Asplund K, Åström T. Psychosocial function and life satisfaction after stroke. Stroke 23:527–531, 1992.

16. Swanson B, Cronin-Stubbs D, Sheldon JA. The impact of psychosocial factors and adapting to physical disability. Rehabil Nurs 14:64–68, 1989.

17. Gershkoff AM, Cifu DX, Currie DM, Means KM. Geriatric rehabilitation. Arch Phys Med Rehabil 74:S402–420, 1993.

18. Clark GS, Murray PK. Rehabiltation of the geriatric patient. In: DeLisa JA (ed), Rehabilitation Medicine: Principles and Practice (pp 410–429). Philadelphia: Lippincott, 1990.

11

Models and Outcome of Stroke Rehabilitation

The health-care reform debate has focused the attention of the rehabilitation community on two areas: How rehabilitation is provided, and what outcome rehabilitation achieves. Implicit in the debate is that some type of rehabilitation service is clinically beneficial to the patient with a disability, a point generally accepted by all health-care professionals and third-party payers. The ultimate question that rehabilitation must address in the current market-driven health-care environment is: What constitutes an outcome meaningful enough to compel a third-party payer to pay for it? This chapter discusses methods of delivering rehabilitation care and outcome analysis for stroke rehabilitation.

WHAT Is Rehabilitation?

Rehabilitation is a coordinated program that provides reliable, conscientious, patient-centered restorative care to minimize the impairment, disability, and handicap caused by a particular set of medical conditions. The rehabilitation program must be defined by quality, that ephemeral characteristic incorporating worth, value, excellence, skill, responsibility, competence, and wisdom (Table 11.1). Quality is defined by all who participate in the rehabilitation process, including the stroke survivor and family, the rehabilitation staff, and the payer.

Inpatient Rehabilitation

Acute Comprehensive Inpatient Rehabilitation

This is the classic rehabilitation service in which a variety of experts functioning as a team converge on a disabled patient and the family to provide a highly coordinated program of physical, functional, psychological, and social restoration designed to maximize recovery and minimize impairment, disability, and handicap (see Appendix). This service is provided in freestanding rehabilitation facilities that are licensed as acute-care hospitals or rehabilitation units of general hospitals. Under Medicare rules, the acute rehabilitation program must provide at least three hours of service from at least two of the following three disciplines: physical and occupational therapies and speech-language pathology. In actual practice, the "three-hour rule" often is not followed strictly. In addition, the acute rehabilitation program must provide 24-hour nursing service and intensive physician care.

Subacute Rehabilitation

The term "subacute" came into use in the early 1990s and is not yet consistently defined. *Subacute care* refers to medical services to meet patient needs that require institution-based care after acute hospital discharge. Subacute services include rehabilitation (functional restoration), hospice, skin management/wound care, and intravenous therapy. Subacute services have emerged from the following:

- The "quicker-but-sicker" phenomenon resulting from the implementation of the prospective payment system of 1983 (Diagnosis-Related Groups).
- Service alternatives developed to meet gaps created by shortened acute hospital stays.
- Cost-containment efforts, particularly by managed-care companies, that seek less expensive alternatives to acute care or rehabilitation.

Within rehabilitation, subacute services offer the distinct advantage of a therapy prescription based solely on patient need rather than reg-

TABLE 11.1   Assessing the Quality of Services Provided to the Persons Served, 1995

Principle:
The organization should provide a mechanism for reviewing the quality of the services and individual plans of the persons served. These reviews should provide an opportunity needed changes. This information should be an integral part of the individual and program planning process.

1. There should be a written description of the system used to assess the quality of the services and the individual plans of the persons served.
   Interpretive Guidelines
   1. The assessment of the quality of services provided to the persons served should include:
      • Control of the review process by the organization
      • Use of individual reviewers who carry out professional functions and who may be either internal or external to the organization.
      • Suggestions offered by the reviewers that may or may not be accepted by the team.
2. The reviews should determine whether:
   a. The assessments of the persons served were thorough, complete, and timely.
   b. The goals and objectives were based on the assessment of the person served.
   c. The services provided related to the goals.
   d. The services were provided for an appropriate duration and intensity.
   e. The services produced the desired results in terms of the stated goals of the individual plans of the persons served.
   f. There were unexpected results/complication.
   g. The persons served have been actively involved in planning and making informed choices regarding their individual plans.
3. An individual providing services should not be the only person to review his/her own work.
   Interpretive Guidelines
   3. Those involved in assessing the quality of services should be professional program and/or clinical personnel. A committee is not required to carry out the assessment of the quality of services, but the process may require more than one person if the person performing the assessment is also providing services within the program.
4. Each review should involve a representative sampling which includes current records and records of person discharged within the last quarter.
5. The system should provide for a review to be performed at least semiannually.

ulations (see the previous discussion of the Medicare's "three-hour rule") while preserving the restorative environment. Properly managed, a subacute program can provide a wide range of services that meet needs of patients too weak to participate in an acute rehabilitation program or who have "graduated" from an acute rehabilitation program. Although subacute rehabilitation can serve patients who can also be treated in comprehensive rehabilitation, subacute is seen as a distinctly different service that provides less physician, psychological, and community-focused care than acute rehabilitation. The current licensing procedure for subacute rehabilitation is as a skilled nursing facility, although the length of stay is similar to acute rehabilitation. Given its licensure, subacute rehabilitation taps into the Medicare reimbursement for skilled nursing home days.

Many programs have now named themselves subacute. Because the Joint Commission on the Accreditation of Health Organizations (JCAHO) or Commission on the Accreditation of Rehabilitation Facilities (CARF) standards for subacute rehabilitation are just now emerging, each program must be carefully scrutinized to discover its component parts. Some subacute rehabilitation programs do not provide a restorative environment, whereas others provide an exemplary interdisciplinary or transdisciplinary team approach with a high level of therapy utilization. There are no published outcome studies for subacute rehabilitation or any that compare outcomes achieved in subacute and acute programs. Used appropriately, subacute care provides an additional rehabilitation option to patients with disabilities who do not meet requirements for acute rehabilitation. Unfortunately, many payers choose subacute care over acute rehabilitation for cost-containment purposes rather than clinical need. Current experience shows that most decisions to use acute or subacute services are driven by cost, not patient need.

Transitional Living Centers

Transitional Living Centers (TLC) provide the intensity and coordination of therapy services provided in inpatient rehabilitation without institutional constraints. More often than not, there is significantly reduced nursing or medical intervention at a TLC. Many of these centers provide home and community services. As of the mid-1990s, Medicare does not pay for TLC services; therefore, the majority of stroke survivors are not treated in these settings.

Outpatient Rehabilitation

The stroke survivor may receive outpatient services at an acute hospital, rehabilitation facility, freestanding rehabilitation outpatient center, freestanding clinic, or therapist's office, either as initial or subsequent treatment. Regardless of location, the patient goes to a facility or facilities where therapeutic services—including physical, recreational, and occupational therapies, speech-language pathology; case management; nursing; and/or psychosocial intervention—are provided. If the patient receives service from more than one therapist, the program may offer some degree of coordination. When providers are in different locations, the amount of coordination tends to decrease unless the payer has a strong external case management system in place.

Outpatient programs often function with the same team focus as inpatient programs. Wherever possible there should be a seamless therapeutic linkage between inpatient and outpatient care so that evaluations do not need to be unnecessarily repeated and lessons and strategies learned in the hospital can be transferred to the outpatient staff. Home treatment and transportation services also may be part of the program.

Outpatient services should emphasize community reintegration. The fact that patients must make an effort to get to the facility subsumes a desire and capability to enter and exit a private vehicle. The outpatient program should form a bridge between the institutional setting and the home.

Home Rehabilitation

As the saying goes, "there's no place like home." Many patients and families prefer home treatment for disabling conditions because of familiarity and convenience. Many home health providers, rehabilitation facilities, and acute-care hospitals provide home health care. All comprehensive home health programs utilize registered nurses, therapists, social workers, and aides. Some home health agencies provide case management (usually through nursing or social service) that link these service providers together in something resembling a team; a few home health providers have formal team meetings similar to those seen in both inpatient and outpatient settings.

Rogoff and associates introduced home stroke rehabilitation over 30 years ago. The study reported on 50 hemiplegic patients enrolled in hospital-based multidisciplinary programs. Half the patients demonstrated significant functional improvement, a finding consistent with inpatient models of the day. Advanced age and prolonged time between stroke and start of treatment, left hemiplegia, and lower income correlated negatively with functional improvement.[1]

Portnow et al. describes a model for multidisciplinary home rehabilitation provided by Wellmark Healthcare Services, Inc.[2] The program was designed to substitute for hospital level care (Table 11.2). No assessment of benefit or outcome measures were mentioned in the reference.

WHO Provides Rehabilitation?

Many health-care workers participate in the rehabilitation process. While in the past the focus has been on licensed clinical staff, those strategically involved now include staff from referring institutions, rehabilitation administrators, as well as one of more of the following professionals:

Admissions coordinator	Physical therapist
Aide (in any discipline)	Program manager
Case manager	Psychologist/counselor
Discharge planner	(Rehabilitation) Nurse
Insurance liaison	Respiratory therapist
Marketer	Social worker
Occupational therapist	Speech-language pathologist
Pharmacist	Therapeutic recreation specialist
Physician (physiatrist, neurologist, orthopedic surgeon, primary care)	Vocational counselor

To provide a therapeutic 24-hour learning environment, of course, these specialists' services must revolve around stroke survivors and families needs. Patients should be supported in their rehabilitation efforts through communication (bedside or on daily individualized schedule), reassurance, and encouragement.

TABLE 11.2   Model of Home Rehabilitation

Team Members	Function	Frequency of Interaction
Physicians	Team leader Sets strategy "Coach" to team (including patient) Diagnosis Chooses wisely among treatment alternatives Orders additional tests and services	Not stated
Nurse	Quarterback Assessment Teaching Directs therapy team	Daily
PT/OT/SP	Assess Train Treat Order equipment	< 5 times/week
Social Worker	Assess Crisis intervention Counseling Resource referral	

(Adapted from Portnow J, Kline T, Daly MA, et al. Multidisciplinary home rehabilitation: A practical model. Clin Geriatr Med 7:695–706, 1991.)

HOW Is Rehabilitation Provided?

In most rehabilitation settings, the specialists listed here work as a team. The well-functioning team provides a level of service and degree of excellence greater than the sum of its parts. Effective teams are characterized by mutual respect, trust, and purpose; willingness to change; flexibility; shared responsibility; eagerness to communicate; and individual and corporate accountability. Teams may be (1) *multidisciplinary,* in which a group of experts act with little or no cross-linking of service; (2) *interdisciplinary,* in which a group of experts act with a significant degree of cross-linking yet responsibilities for patient evaluation and treatment are individually focused, usually based on licensure, training, and experience of the practitioners; OR (3) *transdisciplinary,* in which a group of experts acts with a marked degree of cross-linking and where responsibilities for patient evaluation and treatment are widely disseminated.

Teams function informally and formally. Team members often gather to solve a particular problem or focus on a certain area. The solution or plan generated from this meeting should be disseminated to all team members. Team members may also communicate through a log book or e-mail. In rehabilitation, teams meet formally on a periodic basis—usually every one to two weeks in acute settings, every two to four weeks in subacute and outpatient settings—to discuss and plan patient evaluation and treatment ("team conference" or "team rounds"). Team conference styles vary greatly, but usually fall into one of the following four categories:

1. *Hierarchical*—the conference is run by one individual (most often a physician, nurse, or case manager) who calls on others to participate. Communication tends to be between the leader and the others.

2. *Directed*—the conference is less rigid than the previous style with increased interchange among all members. There is still an internal leader who sets the agenda, time frame, and guides decision making.

3. *Facilitated*—similar to a directed conference, but the leader comes from outside the group and acts as a facilitator or arbiter.

4. *Shared*—the conference functions without a formal leader; discussion moves equally from one member to another.

Stroke survivors and their families may participate directly in team conferences. Experience shows, however, that a team conference is often overwhelming to the patient and may inhibit effective communication. It is preferable to prebrief or debrief the team conference discussion with the patient and family.

Whatever the structure, team conferences (which often include the patient, family, external case manager, and payer, in addition to the treating staff) should provide the participants with adequate information to plan the next steps in the rehabilitation process, recognizing time, budgetary, and social factors. Properly executed, the team conference sparks the thinking of the participants so that problems encountered are more easily solved and obstacles managed. Team rounds should be more than a forum for reporting and gathering data; creativity and energy should characterize this process.

WHERE Is Rehabilitation Provided?

Rehabilitation care is provided in acute-care hospitals, acute rehabilitation hospitals and units, skilled nursing facilities, outpatient centers and departments, transitional living or independent living centers/day hospitals, and the home. For years, stroke rehabilitation has been accomplished mostly in comprehensive rehabilitation inpatient facilities. Recently, other facilities have opened to provide wide-ranging services. As such, the location of service has become less important than the type of service provided.

Hopefully, rehabilitation begins in acute-care facilities. A high level of rehabilitative involvement either on the general medical–surgical or specialized (neurology or orthopedic) floors often prevents many complications that would later inhibit functional process. In the best situations, the acute hospital provides conscientious positioning; range-of-motion therapy to prevent contractures; vigorous skin care; proper bowel care to prevent impaction or obstruction; dysphagia training and diet selection to prevent aspiration; hygienic urinary care to minimize the deleterious effects of incontinence and bladder infection, in addition to formal physical, occupational, and speech therapies.

HOW Is Stroke Rehabilitation Provided?

Stroke rehabilitation may be managed by departments/disciplines, programmatically, or through some merger of the two. Traditionally, rehabilitation hospitals have followed a *departmental* structure in managing clinical service. In this model, for example, the Director of Physical Therapy supervises all physical therapy personnel who may work in any one of a number of clinical programs (spinal cord, stroke, outpatient, and so on). The director links with other directors and senior administration through formal networks through which management decisions and program evaluations are accomplished.

Increasingly, rehabilitation hospitals and units have chosen a *programmatic* structure to manage specific clinical programs. In this model, for example, a stroke rehabilitation program manager coordinates all staff who provide stroke care. This manager evaluates and modifies policies and procedures, personnel ("hires and fires"), and service delivery for the stroke rehabilitation "product line." The manager works with other program managers and senior administration to guide overall institutional functions. In many programmatic models, there are no discipline-specific directors. In the *matrix* combination, responsibility for hiring staff and maintaining professional, discipline-specific standards is retained by the directors of each discipline, but program managers provide leadership in program development and evaluation, strategic planning, and interdepartmental coordination.

Matrix models are difficult to manage because job responsibility and boundaries are not rigid. Matrix models, such as those used by The Rehabilitation Institute at Santa Barbara, Magee Rehabilitation Hospital (Philadelphia), and others, allow professionals to:

- Maintain their identity within each discipline.

- Guarantee that standards specific to each discipline are maintained by department heads who are experienced in their respective fields.

- Integrate new staff more easily because they have the support of professionals in their own disciplines.

- Provide a format for team members to become involved in product planning and development that enables hospitals to manage a portfolio of programs.[3]

An example of a matrix model is shown in Figure 11.1.

WHEN Is Rehabilitation Indicated?

Rehabilitation is indicated for disabled patients who have a reasonable certainty of functional improvement. Rehabilitation efforts are best begun soon after a stroke. Garraway et al. report on their experiences in comparing general hospital and neurologic-focused care for acute-care hospital stroke patients. They found that such intervention increased the proportion of patients who returned to functional independence, but that these gains were not maintained at one year.[4,5] The most important variable in their analysis was early introduction of rehabilitation.[6] Delay results in the development of general medical, musculoskeletal, and neurologic complications—pneumonia, contractures, and spasticity—that inhibit ongoing recovery. Yet many patients who have developed these problems can benefit from a rehabilitation

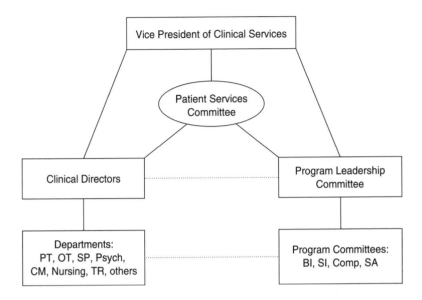

FIGURE 11.1 *Departmental and programmatic responsibilities matrix developed by The Rehabilitation Institute at Santa Barbara.*

program months after the initial stroke. Additionally, at The Rehabilitation Institute at Santa Barbara, we have found that the patients with hemorrhagic stroke have ongoing recovery that makes long-term rehabilitation particularly important.

Candidacy for acute rehabilitation is often determined by a combination of medical, economic, and social factors. In clinical practice, determination of rehabilitation candidacy and appropriate level of service is more an art than a science. Although the results of elaborate studies detailing positive and negative prognostic signs for successful stroke recovery are valuable, clinicians often find themselves accepting or rejecting patients for stroke rehabilitation based on referral patterns, social milieu, inability to provide needed service in another environment, and patients' resources.

Several landmark studies deserve mention with regard to functional improvement and maintenance of gains after stroke rehabilitation. In 1975, Lehmann et al. demonstrated that functional gains, which could not be attributed merely to spontaneous recovery, resulted from rehabilitation of 114 stroke survivors; moreover, rehabilitation was found to be cost-effective in this analysis.[7] Anderson et al. demonstrated that functional gains made during rehabilitation following stroke were maintained or improved by the majority of stroke survivors 2 to 12 years later.[8]

Community participation was a vital factor in maintaining gains. Superimposed health problems adversely affected function. Anderson et al. reported the usefulness of physical, psychological, and interpersonal assessment to gain long-term positive outcomes after stroke rehabilitation. Their study demonstrated that stroke survivors actually improve more than estimated by rehabilitation providers and argued that stroke rehabilitation is justifiable.[9] Other studies have demonstrated improvement in function with "functional oriented medical care" and rehabilitation.[10] Only a minority of authors feel that rehabilitation has a negligible effect on the functional progress of most stroke patients.[11]

Negative predictors for successful stroke rehabilitation include poor postural control and sitting,[12] advanced age, persistent bowel and bladder incontinence, prolonged hyporeflexia, prior stroke, and visuospatial deficits.[13] In a well-designed study of 79 geriatric first-time stroke patients, Aptaker et al. demonstrated that admission serum albumin correlates with discharge modified Barthel Index scores (MBI) and with improvement in Mobility Subscore and Total MBI score during inpatient rehabilitation. Patients with serum albumin greater than or equal to 2.9 g/dL were likely to develop medical complications while undergoing rehabilitation.[14] Intensive care unit (ICU) prognostication is notoriously unreliable; many stroke patients are very sick initially, but then recover neurologically and functionally to a marked degree. In a study of 97 geriatric patients who required intensive care, Chelluri et al. demonstrated that age alone is not an adequate predictor of long-term survival and quality of life.[15]

Stroke survivors with minimal social and economic support in combination with marked neurologic deficits have a poor prognosis for independent living. Opinions vary as to whether it is appropriate to commit resources for acute rehabilitation of patients who frequently become long-term nursing home residents. Many patients with poor neurologic findings and poor prognostic signs for recovery are good candidates for acute rehabilitation because of a family determined to care for the stroke survivor in the home setting. Sometimes it is important to bring patients to acute rehabilitation who have a poor long-term prognosis for independent living in order to treat intercurrent medical conditions or provide a level of sophistication not available in other settings.

Demographic impairment variables alone or in combination have insufficient strength as prognostic indicators to predict patients' ultimate outcome and place of discharge. Disability measures, such as the Functional Independence Measure (FIM[SM]), have been used to classify patients as to their rehabilitation needs.[16] In 113 consecutive stroke admissions, Oczkowski and Barreca found that the admission FIM score, admission postural staging, and age were the best predictors of outcome disability and place of discharge. This study does not represent the typical patient seen in stroke rehabilitation experiences at The Rehabilitation Institute at Santa Barbara, given the fact that the admission to the rehabilitation unit occurred a median of 52 days after stroke onset. It is unclear whether this prognostic data is useful in a more typical time frame from stroke to rehabilitation admission of about one week. What is clear is that ability to live by oneself has less to do with impairment or achieving independent living than with financial and social security.

Goal Setting

Any stroke rehabilitation program should be goal-oriented. Goals need to be defined by the patient, family, payer, and treatment team. These objectives should be specific to the stroke survivor, practical given the medical and neurologic condition of the patient, and possible given the resources and time allotted. In the best situation, the goals drive the type of rehabilitation service provided and the amount of therapy provided; in practice, unfortunately, the skills of the treators may dictate the goals set. Most stroke survivors present with deficits in one or more of the following areas: mobility, self-care, activities of daily living, cognition, communication, continence, swallowing/nutrition, emotional state, social needs, and reintegration (Figure 11.2). Every effort should be made to individualize the patient's program and respect the survivor's desires within these general areas.

Ozer provides a nice model of goal setting, viewing rehabilitation as a place where resourcefulness is generated. To that end, he seeks to develop problem-solving and organizational skills in stroke survivors.[17] He developed five levels of participation between the patient

Pt. Name:								Pt. Present? Y N	Date: / /	☐ Intro	☐ Interim	☐ Discharge

Medical Status		Precautions: __Infections__ __Seizure __Aspiration __Cardiac __Fall __Ortho __Dysreflexia __Bleeding __Code Green
Social/Family/ Discharge Planning		MET GOALS: Y N
Psychologic Adjustment		
Physical Disabilities		

	Profound	Sev	Mod-Sev	Mod	Mild-Mod	Mild	WNL	STG	LTG	COMMENTS
Cognitive										
Perceptual										
Com-muni-cation Exp										
Rec										

	D	Max A	Mod A	Min A	S	Mod I	I			
Rolling										
Sup to Sit										
Transfers										
sit-stand										
level										
unlevel										
toilet										
bath/shower										
car										
Wheelchair										
level										
unlevel/ramp										
parts										
Gait										
level										
unlevel										
curbs										
stairs										
Community										
Eating										
task										
swallow Texture			Strategies							
nutrition										
medications										
Hygiene										
orofacial										
toilet										
sponge bath										
bath/shower										
Bladder continence: day			night							
Bowel continence: day	night		Regularity		Program					
Dressing										
UBD										
LBD										
shoes/brace										
Homemaking										
Meal prep										
Financial										
Leisure										
Driving										
D/C Equipment										
Training										

The Rehabilitation Institute at Santa Barbara
TEAM CONFERENCE

FIGURE 11.2   *Goal Worksheet developed by The Rehabilitation Institute at Santa Barbara.*

and physician (or clinician or rehabilitation team). As the patient ascends to independent participation, she or he moves from compliance with prescribed orders to asking independent questions that can be answered on her or his own; conversely the physician moves from prescription to resource person to facilitator.

Team Goals/Discussion/Treatment Planning	- Home Eval needed Y N
	- Daily living trial date ___/___/___
1. Patient Issues:	- Therapeutic community eval date ___/___/___
2. Obstacles to discharge:	
3. Priorities for achieving next level of care:	
4. Strategies to maximize performance:	

```
                    TEAM MEMBER SIGNATURES              DATE

            Physician _____      ___ /___ /___
        Case Manager _____      ___ /___ /___
 Counselor/Psychologist _____    ___ /___ /___
               Nurse _____      ___ /___ /___
 Occupational Therapy _____      ___ /___ /___
     Physical Therapy _____      ___ /___ /___
Therapeutic Recreation _____     ___ /___ /___
Speech/Language Pathology _____  ___ /___ /___
                     _____      ___ /___ /___
                     _____      ___ /___ /___
                     _____      ___ /___ /___

                    OTHER ATTENDEES

                     _____      ___ /___ /___
                     _____      ___ /___ /___
```

The Rehabilitation Institute at Santa Barbara
TEAM CONFERENCE

FIGURE 11.2   *continued*

Outcome

The patient, family, treatment staff, rehabilitation administrator, payer, and referring physician or system usually define outcome from different perspectives, often resulting in confusion in describing the effectiveness, benefits, and success of stroke rehabilitation. There are many different ways to measure outcome including neurologic status, functional capacity, discharge location, length of stay (inpatient) or service (outpatient), cost/charges of stay, burden of care/time spent providing care, and customer satisfaction (Figure 11.3). We believe that each type of measure represents one face of the multifaceted nature of stroke rehabilitation outcome.

Most stroke rehabilitation programs do not focus on improvement in neurologic status as a measure of success, perhaps because stroke rehabilitation has never been shown to have a demonstrable effect on neurologic recovery.[18] Despite this lack of documentation, stroke rehabilitation limits physical and medical co-morbidities that complicate stroke, thereby allowing maximal neurologic healing. In addition, stroke rehabilitation provides avenues to minimize adverse consequences of incomplete neurologic return, such as spasticity and contractures, that in themselves can cause additional disability. Although researchers may never be able to prove through a well-designed, large-scale study that stroke rehabilitation improves neurologic status and maximizes chances for neurologic return, it is important to monitor neurologic status during stroke rehabilitation. Impairment measures include the standard neurologic examination (mental status, cranial nerve, motor, sensory, reflexes, cerebellar, and gait) and the National Institutes of Health (NIH) Stroke Scale (Table 11.3). Currently, this scale is used most frequently in gauging success of various interventions for acute stroke.[19]

Truncal stability, upper-extremity function, bowel and bladder continence, presenting functional severity, and neuropsychological status represent key prognostic determinants of ultimate functional status. In contrast, home discharge depends more on demographic and socioeconomic characteristics such as age, sex, educational level, and marital status.[20] Functional outcome measures include the Barthel Index (Table 11.4) and the PULSES Profile (Table 11.5), the Katz ADL Scale (Table 11.6) and Evaluation Form (Figure 11.4), and the Functional Independence Measure (Figure 11.5). All have proven reliability in measuring disability after stroke. The FIM was developed to replace the Barthel Index.

Length of stay (LOS) is a useful measure, particularly for third-party payers who relate this variable to per diem cost. Length of stay is only a good indicator when cost is determined on a daily rather than aggregate or case basis. Over the past decade, LOS for acute inpatient stroke rehabilitation has declined to a nationwide average of

PATIENT SATISFACTION SURVEY

Dear Patient,

We at The Rehabilitation Institute at Santa Barbara want to continue to provide the best service possible. We believe that our patients and their families are the best people to evaluate our service performance. Please indicate how well we performed in the categories listed below, and return the form to us. We value your feedback.

	Poor	Fair	Good	Very Good	Excellent
ADMISSION PROCESS — How pleased were you with ...					
1. The admission procedure. Was it timely and efficient?	☐	☐	☐	☐	☐
2. The way our staff informed you about your rehabilitation program?	☐	☐	☐	☐	☐
ROOM — How satisfied were you with ...					
1. The cleanliness of your room?	☐	☐	☐	☐	☐
2. The comfort and temperature?	☐	☐	☐	☐	☐
DIET AND MEALS — How pleased were you with ...					
1. Food preparation, temperature and presentation, (whether or not you were on a special diet)?	☐	☐	☐	☐	☐
MEDICAL CARE — How satisfied were you with ...					
1. How well the physician kept you informed about your rehab program?	☐	☐	☐	☐	☐
2. Your physician's response to your questions and concerns?	☐	☐	☐	☐	☐
3. The level of professionalism and sensitivity shown by the medical staff?	☐	☐	☐	☐	☐

REHAB SERVICES — Please evaluate the care and education that you received from the following services:

	CARE					EDUCATION				
1. Case Management	☐	☐	☐	☐	☐	☐	☐	☐	☐	☐
2. Laboratory	☐	☐	☐	☐	☐	☐	☐	☐	☐	☐
3. Nursing	☐	☐	☐	☐	☐	☐	☐	☐	☐	☐
4. Nutritional Services	☐	☐	☐	☐	☐	☐	☐	☐	☐	☐
5. Occupational Therapy	☐	☐	☐	☐	☐	☐	☐	☐	☐	☐
6. Pharmacy	☐	☐	☐	☐	☐	☐	☐	☐	☐	☐
7. Physical Therapy	☐	☐	☐	☐	☐	☐	☐	☐	☐	☐
8. Psychology/Counseling	☐	☐	☐	☐	☐	☐	☐	☐	☐	☐
9. Radiology	☐	☐	☐	☐	☐	☐	☐	☐	☐	☐
10. Respiratory	☐	☐	☐	☐	☐	☐	☐	☐	☐	☐
11. Speech Therapy	☐	☐	☐	☐	☐	☐	☐	☐	☐	☐
12. Therapeutic Recreation	☐	☐	☐	☐	☐	☐	☐	☐	☐	☐
13. Transportation	☐	☐	☐	☐	☐	☐	☐	☐	☐	☐
14. Volunteer Services	☐	☐	☐	☐	☐	☐	☐	☐	☐	☐

DISCHARGE

1. How well did the team prepare you for your discharge & follow-up care?   ☐ ☐ ☐ ☐ ☐
2. Were you satisfied with your follow-up care?   ☐ ☐ ☐ ☐ ☐

CUSTOMER SERVICE — Please let us know ...

1. If you received a follow-up call, did you find it beneficial?   ☐ ☐ ☐ ☐ ☐
   If yes, how? _____
2. Were you treated with courtesy and respect during your stay?   ☐ ☐ ☐ ☐ ☐
3. What services not available at the Rehabilitation Institute would have been beneficial to you during your stay? _____
4. Do you have any additional comments? _____
_____
_____

The Rehabilitation Institute
AT SANTA BARBARA

Name (optional) _____ M/F ____ Ward ____

Reason for admission (diagnosis) _____

Date you left the Rehabilitation Institute _____   *Thank you for your assistance.*

427 Camino del Remedio, Santa Barbara, CA 93110 805 683-3788

FIGURE 11.3   *Patient Satisfaction Survey form developed by The Rehabilitation Institute at Santa Barbara.*

TABLE 11.3   NIH Stroke Scale

Deficit Tested	Possible Points
Level of Consciousness (LOC)	0–3
LOC questions	0–2
LOC commands	0–2
Gaze abnormally	0–2
Visual loss	0–3
Facial weakness	0–3
Motor weakness in arm	0–4 (right, left)
Motor weakness in leg	0–4 (right, left)
Limb ataxia	0–2
Sensory loss	0–2
Aphasia	0–3
Dysarthria	0–2
Extinction and inattention	0–2
Distal motor function in hand	0–2 (right, left)

(Adapted from Wityk RJ, Pessin MS, Kaplan RF, et al. Serial assessment of acute stroke using the NIH Stroke Scale. Stroke 25:362-365, 1994.)

approximately 24 days—a drop that is expected to continue into the twenty-first century. As capitation and other reimbursement arrangements become more common for rehabilitation, however, LOS will become less useful as an outcome measure. In many facilities, LOS is managed through *critical pathways*—time-driven standards that prompt the rehabilitation team to begin or implement certain treatment at set times. In this sense, length-of-stay assessment can be a valuable clinical tool.

Keith et al. retrospectively compared acute and subacute rehabilitation for stroke.[21] Of the patients studied, 331 received traditional, comprehensive medical rehabilitation averaging 4.92 hours of therapy per day; 97 patients received less intensive subacute services averaging 2.62 hours of therapy per day. Both patient groups were similar in demographics and FIM scores except that at admission the subacute patients had significantly more sphincter control. The total treatment charges were $41,129 for acute and $18,129 for subacute. Compared to subacute patients, acute patients made significantly more functional gains in all areas except communication and social cogni-

TABLE 11.4   Barthel Index

	With Help	Independent
1. Feeding (if food needs to be cut up = help)	5	10
2. Moving from wheelchair to bed and return (includes sitting up in bed)	5–10	15
3. Personal toilet (wash face, comb hair, shave, clean teeth)	0	5
4. Getting on and off toilet (handling clothes, wipe, flush)	5	10
5. Bathing self	0	5
6. Walking on level surface (or, if unable to walk, propel wheelchair)	10	15
*score only if unable to walk	0*	5*
7. Ascend and descend stairs	5	10
8. Dressing (includes tying shoes, fastening fasteners)	5	10
9. Controlling bowels	5	10
10. Controlling bladder	5	10

A patient scoring 100 BI points is continent, feeds herself or himself, dresses herself or himself, gets up out of bed and chairs, bathes unassisted, walks at least a block, and can ascend and descend stairs. This does not mean that he or she is able to live alone: Such a person may not be able to cook, keep house, and meet the public, but is able to get along without attendant care.

tion, but the proportion of patients discharged to the community varied little. The authors noted that the functional status gains of acute rehabilitation might translate into greater long-term benefit in terms of personal competence and less health-care utilization, but there are no data to support or reject that hypothesis. The work of Keith et al. supports the experience of many rehabilitation facilities that have noticed a decline in referral for acute rehabilitation in preference for subacute services.

Feigenson et al., also retrospectively, analyzed medical variables that affect LOS. They found that severe weakness at admission, long interval to rehabilitation admission, severe perceptual or cognitive dysfunction, or homonymous hemianopsia in addition to a motor deficit were related to LOS, whereas age, swallowing difficulties, hemisensory deficit in addition to weakness or certain medical problems were not.[22] In a follow-up study, they found that medical and social screening prior to rehabilitation admission did not reduce LOS,

TABLE 11.5   PULSES Profile

P— Physical condition includes diseases of the viscera (cardiovascular, gastrointestinal, urologic, and endocrine) and neurologic disorders:

1. Medical problems sufficiently stable that medical or nursing monitoring is not required more often than at 3-month intervals.
2. Medical or nurse monitoring is needed more often than at 3-month intervals but not each week.
3. Medical problems are sufficiently unstable as to require regular medical and/or nursing attention at least weekly.
4. Medical problems require intensive medical and/or nursing attention at least daily (excluding personal care assistance only).

U—Upper-limb functions include self-care activities (drink/feed, dress upper/lower, brace/prosthesis, groom, wash, perineal care) dependent mainly on upper-limb function:

1. Independent in self-care without impairment of upper limbs.
2. Independent in self-care with some impairment of upper limbs.
3. Dependent on assistance or supervision in self-care with or without impairment of upper limbs.
4. Dependent totally in self-care with marked impairment of upper limbs.

L— Lower-limb functions include mobility (transfer chair/toilet/tub or shower, walk, stairs, wheelchair) dependent mainly on lower-limb function:

1. Independent in mobility without impairment of lower limbs.
2. Independent in mobility with some impairment in lower limbs such as needing ambulatory aids, a brace or prosthesis, or else fully independent in a wheelchair without significant architectural or environmental barriers.
3. Dependent on assistance or supervision in mobility with or without impairment of lower limbs, or partly independent in a wheelchair, or there are significant architectural or environmental barriers.
4. Dependent totally in mobility with marked impairment of lower limbs.

S— Sensory components include relating to communication (speech and hearing) and vision:

1. Independent in communication and vision without impairment.
2. Independent in communication and vision with some impairment such as mild dysarthria, mild aphasia or need for eyeglasses or hearing aid, or needing regular eye medication.
3. Dependent on assistance, an interpreter, or supervision for communication or vision.
4. Dependent totally for communication or vision.

TABLE 11.5 *continued*

E— Excretory functions (bladder and bowel):
   1. Complete voluntary control of bladder and bowel sphincters.
   2. Control of sphincters allows normal social activities despite urgency or need for catheter, appliances, suppositories, etc. Able to care for needs without assistance.
   3. Dependent on assistance in sphincter management or else has accidents occasionally.
   4. Frequent wetting or soiling from incontinence of bladder or bowel sphincters.

S— Support factors to consider include intellectual and emotional adaptability, support from family unit, and financial ability:
   1. Able to fulfill usual roles and perform customary tasks.
   2. Must make some modification in usual roles and performance of customary tasks.
   3. Dependent on assistance, supervision, encouragement or assistance from a public or private agency because of any of the above considerations.
   4. Dependent on long-term institutional care (chronic hospitalization, nursing home, etc.) excluding time-limited hospital for specific evaluation, treatment, or active rehabilitation.

PULSES Total: Best Score is 6; Worst Score is 24.

(Adapted from Granger CV, Albrecht GL, Hamilton BB. Outcome of comprehensive medical rehabilitation, measurement by PULSES profile and Barthel Index. Arch Phys Med Rehabil 60:145–154, 1979.)

but did improve functional outcome in stroke survivors with perceptual compromise. This finding reinforces the present author's view that LOS is a complex phenomenon based on patient characteristics, neurologic and medical status, psychosocial and economic supports, referral preference, utilization criteria, and third-party payer desires.

There has been a renewed effort to define burden of care/time of care as an outcome measure in stroke rehabilitation. As Disler et al. note, "accurate estimation of the amount of care needed to support a person with a disability in the community is of critical importance."[23] They demonstrated that the FIM and Edinburgh Rehabilitation Status Scale were both reliable predictors of the hours of physical assistance needed; however, neither measure (or any other common one) projected hours of supervision ("hands off") needed.

TABLE 11.6 Katz Activities of Daily Living Scale

The Index of Independence in ADL is based on an evaluation of the functional independence of patients in bathing, dressing, going to toilet, transferring, continence, and feeding.

A	Independent in feeding, continence, transferring, going to toilet, dressing and bathing
B	Independent in all but one of these functions
C	Independent in all but bathing and one additional function
D	Independent in all but bathing, dressing, and one additional function
E	Independent in all but bathing, dressing, going to toilet, and one additional function
F	Independent in all but bathing, dressing, going to toilet, transferring, and one additional function
G	Dependent in all six functions
Other	Dependent in at least two functions but not classifiable as C, D, E, or F

(Adapted from Katz S, Ford AB, Moskowitz RW, et al. Studies of illness in the aged. The index of ADL: A standardized measure of biological and psychosocial function. JAMA 185(12):914–919, 1963. Used with permission.)

Future investigation of stroke and its rehabilitation efforts must become more sophisticated in order to determine the benefits of intervention. The Task Forces on Stroke Impairment, Disability, and Handicap made the following recommendations for all future stroke outcome research: Studies should measure time from onset; specify laterality of brain lesion, not peripheral manifestations; and use the same neuroimaging technique for all cases. Although the Disability Task Force did not endorse any specific functional instrument, the scale(s) used should include mobility, self-care, sphincter control, communication, cognition, behavior, leisure, quality of life, and complex task assessment. In addition, the Task Force recommended other outcome factors such as living arrangement, place of residence, utilization of health-care resources, ability to work, and change in functional status. Disability should relate to impairments, including co-morbidities and complications, and be measured from onset of stroke and at standard intervals (e.g., 3, 6, and 12 months). The Handicap Task Force recommended a synthesis of current stroke handicap data and development of new research instruments for study of stroke handicap. Future studies should consider context of stroke handicap and degree of

Name: _____   Date of Evaluation: _____

For each area of functioning listed below, check description that applies. (The word "assistance" means supervision, direction or personal assistance)

Bathing—either sponge bath, tub bath, or shower.

☐ Receives no assistance (gets in and out of tub by self if tub is usual means of bathing)

☐ Receives assistance in bathing only one part of the body (such as back or a leg)

☐ Receives assistance in bathing more than one part of the body (or not bathed)

Dressing—gets clothes from closets and drawers, including underclothes, outer garments and using fasteners (including braces if worn).

☐ Gets clothes and gets completely dressed without assistance.

☐ Gets clothes and gets dressed except for assistance in tying shoes.

☐ Receives assistance in getting clothes or in getting dressed, or stays partly or completely undressed.

Toileting—going to the "toilet room" for bowel and urine elimination; cleaning self after elimination, and arranging clothes.

☐ Goes to "toilet room," cleans self, and arranges clothes without assistance (may use object for support such as cane, walker, or wheelchair and may manage night bedpan or commode, emptying same in morning.)

☐ Receives assistance in going to "toilet room" or in cleansing self or in arranging clothes after elimination or in use of night bedpan or commode.

☐ Doesn't go to room termed "toilet" for the elimination process.

Transfer

☐ Moves in and out of bed as well as in and out of chair without assistance (may be using object for support such as cane or walker)

☐ Moves in or out of bed or chair with assistance

☐ Doesn't get out of bed

Continence

☐ Controls urination and bowel movement completely by self

☐ Has occasional "accidents"

☐ Supervision helps keep urine or bowel control; catheter is used, or patient is incontinent.

Feeding

☐ Feeds self without assistance

☐ Feeds self except for getting assistance in cutting meat or buttering bread

☐ Receives assistance in feeding or is fed partly or completely by using tubes or intravenous fluids

FIGURE 11.4   *Katz Index of Independence in Activities of Daily Living Evaluation Form*

(From Katz S, Ford AB, Moskowitz RW, et al. Studies of illness in the aged. The index of ADL: A standardized measure of biological and psychosocial function. JAMA 185(12): 914–919, 1963. Used with permission.)

7 Complete Independence (Timely, Safely) 6 Modified Independence (Device)		NO HELPER

L
E
V
E
L
S
	Modified Dependence
	  5 Supervision
	  4 Minimal Assist (Subject = 75% +)
	  3 Moderate Assist (Subject = 50% +)
	
	Complete Dependence
	  2 Maximal Assist (Subject = 25% +)
	  1 Total Assist (Subject = 0% +)
		HELPER

Self-Care   ADMIT   DISCHG   FOL-UP
A. Eating
B. Grooming
C. Bathing
D. Dressing - Upper Body
E. Dressing - Lower Body
F. Toileting

Sphincter Control
G. Bladder Management
H. Bowel Management

Transfers
I. Bed, Chair, Wheelchair
J. Toilet
K. Tub, Shower

Locomotion
L. Walk/wheelchair   (Walk / Wheelchair / Both)
M. Stairs

Motor Subtotal Score

Communication
N. Comprehension   (Auditory / Visual / Both)
O. Expression   (Vocal / Non-vocal / Both)

Social Cognition
P. Social Interaction
Q. Problem Solving
R. Memory

Cognitive Subtotal Score

Total FIM

NOTE: Leave no blanks; enter 1 if patient not testable due to risk

FIGURE 11.5 *FIM^SM Form*

handicap before and after stroke. Implementation of these recommendations should strengthen the quality, comparability, and usefulness of stroke outcome studies.[24]

Conclusion

The future for stroke rehabilitation is bright. Practitioners need to move forward to develop a more patient-focused approach to stroke care with emphasis on patient-determined goals and ownership of the rehabilitation process, patient-centered cost-reduction strategies, continuous quality improvement, outcome focus, and paradigm pliancy.[25] In the next decade, increased efforts must be made to limit initial damage from stroke, prevent future stroke and medical complications of stroke, implement practice parameters and standards to reduce variability of treatment, and provide insurance coverage for all who suffer stroke.[26]

References

1. Rogoff JB, Cooney DV, Kutner B. Hemiplegia: A study of home rehabilitation. J Chronic Dis 17:539–550, 1964.
2. Portnow J, Kline T, Daly MA, et al. Multidisciplinary home rehabilitation: A practical model. Clin Geriatr Med 7:695–706, 1991.
3. Sterthouse LM. Support by synergy. Rehab Manage (Dec/Jan): 56–62, 1993.
4. Garraway WM, Jakhtar AJ, Prescott RJ, et al. Management of acute stroke in the elderly: Preliminary results of a controlled trial. BMJ 281:1040–1043, 1980.
5. Garraway WM, Jakhtar AJ, Prescott RJ, et al. Management of acute stroke in the elderly: Follow-up of a controlled trial. BMJ 281:827–829, 1980.
6. Smith ME, Garraway WM, Smith DL, et al. Therapy impact on functional outcome in a controlled trial of stroke rehabilitation. Arch Phys Med Rehabil 63:21–24, 1982.
7. Lehmann JF, DeLateur BJ, Fowler RS, et al. Stroke: Does rehabilitation affect outcome? Arch Phys Med Rehabil 56:375–383, 1975.
8. Anderson E, Anderson TP, Kottke FJ. Stroke rehabilitation: Maintenance of achieved gains. Arch Phys Med Rehabil 58:345–352, 1977.
9. Anderson TP, McClure WJ, Athelstan G, et al. Stroke rehabilitation: Evaluation of its quality by assesssing patient outcomes. Arch Phys Med Rehabil 59:170–175, 1978.
10. Feldman DJ, Lee PR, Unterecker JA, et al. Comparison of functionally orientated medical care and formal rehabilitation in the management of

patients with hemiplegia due to cerebrovascular disease. J Chronic Dis 15:297–310, 1962.

11. Lind KA. Synthesis of studies on stroke rehabilitation. J Chronic Dis 35:133–149, 1982.

12. Sandin KJ, Smith BS. The measure of balance in sitting in stroke rehabilitation prognosis. Stroke 21:82–86, 1990.

13. Jongbloed L. Prediction of function after stroke: A critical review. Stroke. 17:765–776, 1986.

14. Aptaker RL, Roth EJ, Reichhardt G, et al. Serum albumin level as a predictor of geriatric stroke rehabilitation. Outcome 75:80–84, 1994.

15. Chelluri L, Pinsky MR, Donahoe MP, et al. Long-term outcome of critically ill elderly patients requiring intensive care. JAMA 269:3119–3123, 1993.

16. Oczkowski WJ, Barreca S. The Functional Independence Measure: Its use to identify rehabilitation needs in stroke survivors. Arch Phys Med Rehabil 74:1291–1299, 1993.

17. Ozer MN: Involving people with stroke in their care. Adv Rehabil (June): 98, 1995.

18. Wood-Dauphinee SL, Shapiro S, Bass E, et al. A randomized trial of team care following stroke. Stroke 15:864, 1984.

19. Wityk RJ, Pessin MS, Kaplan RF, et al. Serial assessment of acute stroke using the NIH Stroke Scale. Stroke 25:362–365, 1994.

20. Stineman MG, Granger CV. Epidemiology of stroke-related disability and rehabilitation outcome. In: Goldberg G (ed), Stroke Rehabilitation. Physical Medicine and Rehabilitation Clinics of North America, vol 2 (pp 457–471). Philadelphia: Saunders, 1991.

21. Keith RA, Wilson DB, Gutierrez P. Acute and subacute rehabilitation for stroke: A comparison. Arch Phys Med Rehabil 76:495–500, 1995.

22. Feigenson JS, McDowell FH, Meese P, et al. Factors influencing outcome and length of stay in a stroke rehabilitation unit. Stroke 8:651–663, 1977.

23. Disler PB, Roy CW, Smith BP. Predicting hours of care needed. Arch Phys Med Rehabil 74:139-143, 1993.

24. Task Force on Stroke Impairment, Task Force on Stroke Disability, and Task Force on Stroke Handicap. Symposium Recommendations for Methodology in Stroke Outcome Research. In: Gresham GE (ed), Methodologic Issues in Stroke Outcome Research. Stroke 21(suppl II):II-68–II-73, 1990.

25. Burgess C. The New Rehabilitation Paradigm. Lakewood, CA: Connie Burgess and Associates, 1993.

26. NSA. Be Stroke Smart. 10th Anniversary Newsletter 11:16-17, 1994.

APPENDIX

CARF STANDARDS FOR COMPREHENSIVE
INPATIENT REHABILITATION, 1995

Program Description

A Comprehensive Inpatient program is a 24-hour program of coordinated and integrated medical and rehabilitation services.

The following three categories describe the types of Comprehensive Inpatient programs for which organizations may seek accreditation. When applying for accreditation an organization, depending on how it is licensed in the state where it is located, should indicate the categories in which it is seeking accreditation. Dependent upon the licenses held, an organization may choose to be accredited in any or all of the three categories. The organization should also indicate whether it wishes to be designated as a pediatric program in any or all of the three categories.

CATEGORY ONE: Hospital

This program of acute rehabilitation is located in an organization that is licensed as a hospital. The persons served have expected outcomes of returning to the community with or without support or of progressing to another level of rehabilitation care—e.g., outpatient, home health, etc. The persons served in Category One have the following characteristics:

1. Are at high risk of potential medical instability.

2. Receive regular, direct individual contact by rehabilitation physicians determined by their medical and rehabilitation needs.

3. Have multiple and/or complex rehabilitation nursing needs and a potential for needing high medical acuity skilled nursing.

4. Based on their individual needs, receive a daily minimum of three hours of services a minimum of five days per week from the interdisciplinary team, which includes an occupational therapist, a physical therapist, a psychologist, a social worker, a speech-language pathologist, and a therapeutic recreation specialist.

5. Have education and training opportunities for themselves as well as family members on an ongoing basis.

Examples of persons served in Category One are individuals with diagnoses including, but not limited to, cerebral vascular accidents, neuromuscular diseases, multiple traumas, spinal cord injuries, and brain injuries.

CATEGORY TWO: Hospital
Hospital-Based Skilled Nursing Facility
Skilled Nursing Facility

This program of subacute rehabilitation is located in an organization that is licensed as a hospital, a hospital-based skilled nursing facility, or a skilled nursing facility. The persons served have expected outcomes of returning home or progressing to another level of rehabilitation care—e.g., Comprehensive Inpatient Category One, outpatient, home health, etc. The persons served in Category Two have the following characteristics:

1. Have a variable risk of potential medical instability.

2. Have regular, direct individual contact by rehabilitation physicians determined by their medical and rehabilitation needs.

3. Have multiple and/or complex rehabilitation nursing needs and a potential for needing high medical acuity skilled nursing.

4. Based on their individual needs, receive a daily minimum of one hour of services a minimum of five days per week from the interdisciplinary team, which includes an occupational therapist, a physical therapist, a psychologist, a social worker, a speech-language pathologist, and a therapeutic recreation specialist.

5. Have education and training opportunities for themselves as well as family members on an ongoing basis.

Examples of persons served in Category Two are individuals with diagnoses including, but not limited to, cerebral vascular accidents, neuromuscular diseases, brain injuries, orthopedic conditions, and multiple traumas.

CATEGORY THREE: Hospital-based Skilled Nursing Facility
Skilled Nursing Facility

This program of subacute rehabilitation is located in an organization that is licensed as a hospital-based skilled nursing facility or a skilled nursing facility. The persons served have an expected outcome of returning to the community (e.g., home or board and care) with or without support as needed. The persons served in this category have the following characteristics:

1. Are at low risk of potential medical instability.

2. Have regular, direct individual contact by rehabilitation physicians determined by their medical and rehabilitation needs.

3. Have routine rehabilitation nursing needs and a low risk of needing high medical acuity skilled nursing.

4. Based on their individual needs, receive a daily minimum of one to three hours of services a minimum of five days per week from the interdisciplinary team, which includes an occupational therapist, a physical therapist, a psychologist, a social worker, a speech-language pathologist, and a therapeutic recreation specialist.

5. Have education and training opportunities for themselves as well as family members on an ongoing basis.

Examples of persons served in Category Three are individuals with diagnoses including, but not limited to, orthopedic conditions (e.g., uncomplicated total hip replacements or total knee replacements), amputations, and multiple traumas without complications.

(From Medical Rehabilitation, Section 5.A [pp 83–85]. Used with permission of the Commission on Accreditation of Rehabilitation Facilities, Tucson, AZ.)

12

Case Studies

This chapter follows the clinical course of five composite patients with different types of stroke. Use of a case study format, we hope, should better cement understanding of this book and demonstrate the relationship between acute-care management and rehabilitation.

Case One (LK): Intracerebellar Hemorrhage

A 55-year-old, known alcoholic, right-handed white man was brought to the emergency department (ED) by the police when he was found on the street having difficulty with balance. The patient also complained of difficulty swallowing, change in voice sound, and dizziness. The examination was remarkable—blood pressure 170/86, hepatomegaly, intrinsic foot–muscle atrophy, pain and numbness over the right side of the face, falling to the right, small right pupil, right eyelid droop, decreased gag reflex, and impaired pain sensation over the left side of the body. He could not walk. The initial ED evaluation failed to confirm intoxication; blood work for chemistry, hematology, and coagulation was normal except for elevated liver enzymes. The patient underwent a CT scan which showed an old area of infarction in the left basal ganglion and a right intracerebellar hemorrhage. A neurosurgeon was called and made arrangements to transport the patient to the OR for urgent hematoma evacuation.

The evacuation went well and the patient was brought to the neurosurgical ICU. His alertness improved, but visual and swallowing deficits remained. On postoperative Day 2, PT, consisting of bedside ROM and gradual sitting in bed, was begun. On postoperative Day 3, a rehabilitation consultation was obtained from a physiatrist. She noted dysphagia, dysarthria with a wet-voice quality, fair alertness, memory loss, and loss of self-care and mobility skills. Occupational therapy and SLP services were added. The patient was placed on NPO until a VSS could be accomplished. The patient was transferred to the general hospital floor.

On postoperative Day 4, the patient knew where he was but did not know the circumstances of his hospital admission. The swallowing study showed frank aspiration of thin liquids, vallecular penetration without frank aspiration of thick liquids, and delay in swallow of pureed foods. A percutaneous endoscopic gastrostomy (PEG) tube was placed on postoperative Day 5 without complication. The physiatrist recommended rehabilitation admission, and the patient was transferred to a freestanding rehabilitation hospital on postoperative Day 6.

On presentation at the rehabilitation facility, the examination revealed general improvement in neurologic status, but the patient still complained of dizziness and swallowing problems and evidenced poor coordination on the right upper and lower extremities, falling to right so that he could not stand or walk without maximal assistance, and dysarthria with a wet-voice quality. He participated quickly in all aspects of the examination, which showed poor memory for objects at three minutes. The following focus list was developed:

- Impairment in mobility, characterized by loss of righting response and impulsivity.

- Impairment in cognition, characterized by decreased memory and attention, impulsivity, and poor safety judgment.

- Impairment in self-care/ADLs, with poor coordination of right (dominant) upper extremity, cognitive loss, and impulsivity.

Initially, the mobility treatment plan focused on transfers. It was noted that the patient maintained balance better if he stayed somewhat crouched in transfers; this technique was consistently applied in all settings. Therapeutic exercise included routine strengthening and endurance-building exercises, as well as specific Frankel exercises for coordination. Mirror and verbal cueing were used to provide visual and auditory feedback. After two weeks, the patient gained the ability to transfer on his own but often found himself in potentially unsafe situations. The staff videotaped his transfers and it played back to reinforce self-control.

Memory training began with routine drill-oriented cognitive exercises. Soon, however, the patient's daily routine was incorporated into this training so that he was required to remember his daily schedule and medications. Verbal feedback improved error awareness. A log book was used, but its effectiveness was compromised by incomplete staff entries. Real-life experiences in the community provided concrete information about problem solving, which was surprisingly good in this more natural setting. The diplopia was managed with an eye patch over alternating eyes and with vision therapy.

Two weeks into his stay, when ambulation training commenced, the patient complained of right calf pain. Physical examination showed that everything was entirely normal. The patient was sent for a lower-extremity venous Doppler study which demonstrated an acute right popliteal DVT. The patient was started on intravenous heparin at the rehabilitation hospital and shortly thereafter was switched to oral warfarin, with daily coagulation monitoring. The patient could not bear weight on the affected leg for five days; therapy was performed in bed and with left lower-extremity weight bearing. Once allowed to bear weight again, his activity level picked up where he left off.

Initially, all nutrition came through the feeding tube. The patient reported a weight loss of seven pounds during his acute-care hospitalization. The feeding formula was changed to a higher calorie product that unfortunately caused diarrhea. Judicious swallowing training beginning with pureed food was begun. The SLP checked for worsening of voice quality after each swallow. Once the patient was able to swallow four ounces of pureed food in a treatment session, he was placed in a dysphagia group with three other patients. In two weeks, he was able to take 50 percent of his required calories orally. He was advanced to self-feeding, but was found to need verbal restraint on how to slow down and was very sloppy with food placement. A one-pound weight was placed on his right wrist to improve feeding accuracy. A repeat VSS done three weeks after rehabilitation admission showed minimal radiographic improvement in swallow delay and penetration, though there was no aspiration of thin liquids. The SLP felt that the patient would need long-term gastrostomy supplementation; he was trained in self G-tube feeding, incorporating memory strategies to follow all steps in proper sequence.

The patient was discharged to a alcohol abuse halfway house three and half weeks after rehabilitation admission. He was able to transfer, ambulate, and negotiate six steps alone with a single-point cane. Rudimentary self-care skills were independent, but the patient required assistance for home management. He could feed himself orally or through the feeding tube.

Outpatient services focused on improving gait distance and technique. Gait training followed a similar approach using auditory, visual, and tactile feedback. The patient showed good technique on level, unlevel, smooth, and uneven surfaces quite quickly, requiring a single-point cane for stability.

Case Two (BR): Subarachnoid Hemorrhage

The patient, a 38-year-old right-handed black female with a history of tobacco use and no other medical problems, was brought by her husband to the ER with complaints of two hours' history of severe headache with nausea and one episode of vomiting. Two weeks previously she had had a transient headache associated with slightly slurred speech. In the ED she was alert and conversant initially and was able to describe her pain as the worst headache of her life. Later she became somnolent and disoriented with no localizing neurologic symptoms. Ten minutes later she exhibited a generalized tonic–clonic seizure treated with IV diazepam followed by a loading dose of IV phenytoin.

Vital signs throughout her course in the ED were normal. On examination at the time of her admission, she was noted to have nuchal rigidity with pain on forced neck flexion, disorientation, normal strength in reflex examination, and poor sitting balance. An emergency CT scan was obtained which demonstrated diffuse subarachnoid hemorrhage over the cerebral hemispheres and entering the interhemispheric fissure. Lumbar puncture was performed; a significant number of red blood cells were noted in both tube one and tube four.

The patient was admitted to the ICU. That same evening she underwent four-vessel angiography which demonstrated an anterior communicating artery aneurysm. Neurosurgical consultation was obtained and an intracranial pressure monitoring device was placed. The patient was taken to OR and underwent clipping of her aneurysm. She was treated prophylactically against vasospasm with nimodipine. Initially she did well postoperatively, but on Day 2, she developed abrupt onset right hemiparesis. Transcranial Doppler ultrasonography was indicative of severe spasm of the left MCA and the patient continued to be treated aggressively in the ICU setting. She required tube feeding via NG tube secondary to lethargy. Her intracranial pressure remained within the normal range throughout her course and her monitor was removed on hospital Day 5. She was eventually stabilized and transferred to the floor where she continued to show improvement in neurologic function. A rehabilitation consultation was obtained, and on hospital Day 10, she was transferred to the rehabilitation facility.

On admission to that facility some deficits were noted. She actually did quite well on a dysphagia evaluation and was cleared to start a pureed diet with thick liquids; however, her NG tube was maintained pending evaluation of her PO intake. She was noted to have moderate right hemiparesis with hyperreflexia and four beats of clonus at the ankle. She had a very mild expressive aphasia but her receptive language capabilities were intact. She had no significant visual field cut or dysarthria. The following focus list was generated:

- Impairment in swallowing: It was felt that the patient would advance rather quickly to purely oral feeding but the NG tube was maintained secondary to concerns of adequate food intake.

- Impairment in self-care, secondary to right upper-extremity paresis.

- Impairment in mobility, secondary to decreased balance reactions in sitting and right-sided weakness.

- Seizure disorder: The patient was to be changed from phenytoin to carbamazepine for seizure treatment.

The patient rapidly advanced to adequate fluid intake of 1500 ml per day and her NG tube was pulled on rehabilitation hospital Day 3. She continued to improve and within two weeks of her arrival in rehabilitation was taking in a mechanical soft diet with thin liquids; speech therapy for dysphagia was discontinued.

The patient's ability to participate in self-care was soon limited by increasing right upper-extremity shoulder pain. Although she had good distal function of her right upper extremity, she had a two-finger subluxation of her right shoulder at admission and this gradually became more and more painful with the return of spasticity and some muscle imbalance around the right shoulder. This was managed by using a lapboard, which helped support her shoulder during sitting, and she wore a sling during ambulation. She was, however, able to master the hemitechnique of dressing rather rapidly. She made good progress in her self-care.

With respect to mobility, she had significant problems with spasticity in both the upper and lower extremities with clonus interfering with gait training. She was treated initially with baclofen 5 mg tid with some gradual improvement. Once the dose was increased to 10 mg tid, she became somewhat somnolent. Because of the change in her mental status, a CT scan of the head, which demonstrated an expansion in the size of her ventricles from her previous scan, was obtained. She was transferred back to acute care where a neurosurgeon placed a ventricular peritoneal shunt.

She returned to rehabilitation on postoperative Day 4 at which time the baclofen was restarted and she again became somnolent. At that point baclofen was discontinued and dantrolene was begun which helped decrease her tone without an increase in somnolence. Her liver function tests were monitored throughout the rest of her hospitalization and remained stable. She was able to attain a level of modified independence with gait and transfers after a four-week LOS.

She had no further seizure activity during her rehabilitation stay. She was started on carbamazepine 200 mg qid with a gradual increase in her dose; and when the carbamazepine level was at a near therapeutic level, her phenytoin was tapered and then eventually discontinued. She maintained adequate levels of carbamazepine with no further seizure activity. Liver function tests did not show any elevation. She did have a decrease in her white blood cell count which was followed on a weekly basis but no significant neutropenia was noted. Aside from the development of hydrocephalus, the only other medical complication this patient experienced was a urinary tract infection which was treated with appropriate antibiotics and resolved.

Her shoulder pain was managed initially with mechanical devices such as slings and lapboards. Approximately two weeks into her hospitalization she developed exquisite tenderness across the mesacarpophalangeal joints of her right hand with continued shoulder pain. At that time, a clinical diagnosis of reflex sympathetic dystrophy was made and she was treated with a methylprednisolone and VE contrast baths with near total resolution of her symptoms.

The patient did very well in her rehabilitation program and was discharged home at a modified-independent level. Her husband was retired from the military and thus was available to supervise the patient in all areas, as well as to transport her back and forth to PT by car. She made good progress in her outpatient therapy program and after a course of vocational rehabilitation was able to return to her job as a data entry clerk and resumed most of her household duties. She continued to be restricted with respect to driving secondary to DMV rules. With adequate seizure-control medication, she resumed driving one year after her event.

Case Three (TZ): Cardioembolic Left MCA Stroke

This patient, a 68-year-old right-handed Asian man with a history of hypertension and coronary artery disease characterized by stable angina, was brought to the ER by paramedics after his wife found him at home weak and unable to get up. She returned after running some errands to find him on the ground with urinary incontinence; he was unable to speak. She had difficulty arousing him. Blood pressure on presentation was 200/100; initial examination showed a patient with a left-gaze preference and obvious right-sided weakness. Tone and reflexes were diminished on the right. He was unable to follow commands or produce any verbalization though he did vocalize a response to pain.

Telemetry revealed an irregularly irregular heartbeat with a 12-lead EKG showing atrial fibrillation with a rapid ventricular response rate of 120. He also had nonspecific ST wave changes. Routine laboratories were remarkable for mild hypokalemia with a potassium of 3.4 and mild elevation in his BUN and creatinine. A noncontrast CT was obtained which showed no bleed but did hint at effacement of the left temporal parietal sulci with mild left-to-right shift. It also revealed a small area of previous infarction in the right basal ganglia. The patient was admitted to the telemetry unit and was digitalized with prompt decrease in his ventricular response rate. He was made NPO secondary to concerns about dysphagia.

Initially, the patient was quite lethargic. He was started on low-flow O_2. MI was ruled out by serial EKGs and cardiac enzymes. Dysphagia evaluation done by a speech therapist on hospital Day 2 recommended NPO status secondary to poor level of alertness. He had a follow-up CT scan on hospital Day 4 which revealed delineation of a left-middle cerebral artery ischemic stroke with some surrounding edema. A transthoracic echocardiogram failed to demonstrate a mural thrombosis; the family declined transesophageal echocardiography.

Dysphagia evaluation was repeated on hospital Day 5 and he was able to tolerate pureed foods and thick liquids. The speech therapist was uncomfortable with advancing his diet further until obtaining a modified barium swallow which was done on hospital Day 6. The study revealed only very mild delay of swallowing reflex and no aspiration so he was upgraded to a mechanical soft diet with thin liquids. However, his oral intake was poor secondary to preferring more familiar ethnic foods that his wife subsequently began to bring in for him. He was stabilized and was transferred to the rehabilitation center. His primary doctor recommended anticoagulation in approximately another week.

At the time of his admission to rehabilitation, he continued to have receptive and expressive aphasia with his only utterances being occasional automatic speech in his native language, Korean. His left-gaze preference had resolved and he did not seem to have any discreet visual field cut. He evidenced right hemiparesis with some emerging tone distally in the hand and some trace movements at the hip and knee in the leg. Sensation appeared impaired on the right side of his body. He was noted by the nursing staff to be incontinent of bowel and had a Foley catheter in place. Significant edema of his right hand also was noted. The following focus list was generated:

- Impairment of mobility, secondary to dense right hemiparesis, impaired sitting balance, and right-sided hemisensory loss.

- Impairment in self-care and ADLs, with severe motor involvement of his dominant extremity. Again, poor sitting balance affected his self-care and ADL abilities.

- Impaired communication, marked by difficulty following one-step commands and complete lack of functional writing, speaking, or reading. He was, however, able to use some gestures effectively.

- Impairment in bowel and bladder function, marked by Foley catheterization and bowel incontinence.

- Right-hand edema.

The patient developed antigravity strength in his hip flexors and the extensors in a pattern of extensor synergy rather rapidly and was able to incorporate this in transfer training. He eventually was able to obtain a level of minimal assist to contact guard with transfers from wheelchair to bed. He had started to ambulate but was still requiring moderate assist to walk with a wide-based quad cane and a rigid ankle AFO at the time of discharge.

The patient was disinterested in self-care therapy, apparently secondary to cultural issues. There was difficulty in getting the family to understand that they should not necessarily help him with all of his self-care. Because there was little motivation within the family unit to foster independence and self-care, it was decided to concentrate more on functional transfers. At the time of his discharge from rehabilitation, he was minimal-to-moderate assist for most self-care but was minimal assist for his functional transfers.

His ability to communicate improved gradually. The first priority of communication was establishing a consistent gesture for needing to use the toilet which was done within the first two weeks. At that point he became continent of bowel once he was able to signal reliably to the nursing staff. He gradually improved in his yes/no reliability, attaining 95 percent for simple questions. He was able to follow motor commands with visual cues accurately for commands containing one or two steps, but broke down with higher-level commands. By the time of discharge, the patient was able to use a picture communication board and was also able to use gestures to make his basic needs known. He was having some return of speech in the form of automatic social speech more consistently in his native Korean than in English. He did not regain functional reading or writing even though he did attain the ability to sign documents with his left hand.

His Foley catheter was removed during the first week of his rehabilitation stay, but he had high postvoid residuals as measured by a bladder volume instrument. His catheter had to be replaced; he had a tendency to pull at it and had significant hematuria requiring irrigation of the catheter. He was started on a trial of terazosin 1 mg at bedtime and his Foley catheter was subsequently removed with residuals in the vicinity of approximately 200 ml. After increasing his dose of terazosin to 2 mg, he was able to void with residuals less than 100 ml.

The patient had significant hand edema at admission. This responded nicely to use of an elasticized glove, ice slurry cooling, and elevation of the hand on a foam wedge placed on his wheelchair lapboard. He also received anti-edema massage, and he and his family were instructed on how to do follow all these maneuvers for fair control of his edema.

The patient's atrial fibrillation was well controlled with digoxin during his hospitalization. After seven days in rehabilitation, he was restarted on warfarin without any difficulties. He had been on subcutaneous heparin for DVT prophylaxis prior to starting the warfarin. The delay in starting the warfarin was secondary to his primary internist's concern about hemorrhagic transformation of his large infarct. He did have an episode of angina during physical therapy. An EKG, which was unchanged from baseline, was obtained, and the episode resolved after two nitroglycerin tablets. He was followed in therapy for several days on telemetry with no significant EKG changes and he had no subsequent anginal episodes.

Early on in his hospitalization, the patient developed significant depression. Because of the language difficulties/barrier, it was difficult for him to communicate his feelings and participate in supportive psychotherapy or group therapy. He was started on sertraline 50 mg daily to which he responded quite nicely; after a short time on the medication, he exhibited less frustration with his speech deficits, participated more enthusiastically in his rehabilitation program, and demonstrated an improved appetite.

The patient was discharged home with his family after his wife was trained to assist him in all areas of care. He attended outpatient therapy eventually obtaining a level of modified independence with gait. His wife continued to assist him in self-care so OT was not really a priority of his outpatient program. He continued in long-term ST but it was soon found to be more effective to have his wife work with him in his native Korean with the direction of the speech therapist. He was eventually able to utter short phrases and make his needs known. He later participated in an adaptive golf program and a stroke exercise group.

Case Four (WS): Right Internal Capsule (Lacunar) Stroke

An 86-year-old Latin American female patient, with a history of hypertension and noninsulin-dependent diabetes mellitus, who noted left-sided weakness, slurred speech, and drooling, was brought by her family to the ER for evaluation. Admission blood pressure was

210/105. Her general physical examination was unremarkable except for cataracts, slight memory loss that her family indicated was her baseline state. She had normal visual fields, a left-central seventh cranial nerve palsy, dysarthria without aphasia, decreased motor movements with poor control of saliva, and complete left hemiplegia other than preservation of left hip flexion at an approximate level of 2/5. Sensation was normal. Routine laboratories were remarkable only for a blood glucose of 246. The initial brain CT showed only age-related atrophy and mild periventricular white matter ischemic changes, so she was admitted to the medical floor.

The patient was made NPO pending a speech evaluation of her swallowing. A carotid duplex was done which showed a 50 percent stenosis of her left internal carotid artery without hemodynamic compromise. She did have some mild plaquing at the bifurcation on the right with no significant stenosis. An echocardiogram was done, which showed mild left ventricular hypertrophy consistent with her long history of hypertension. No valvular abnormalities were noted. She did have some hypokinesias of her inferior wall with an ejection fraction of 45 percent. EKG showed normal sinus rhythm with evidence of an old inferior wall MI and nonspecific ST wave changes.

Initial chest x-ray was negative for any acute cardiopulmonary process. On hospital Day 2, the patient developed a fever to 102°F, wet-vocal quality, and mild tachypnea with a respiratory rate of 28. Oxygen saturation by pulse oximetry was 88 percent on room air so she was started on low-flow O_2. Sputum culture and sensitivity was sent; she was started on IV antibiotics. She remained NPO. On hospital Day 3, a chest x-ray was obtained which revealed an early infiltration in the left-lower lobe that had not been present on her admission film. Speech evaluation of her swallowing found a mildly delayed swallow, wet-vocal quality and she was recommended to remain NPO.

On hospital Day 4, she had an MRI of the brain that showed a small lacunar CVA in the right internal capsule. She responded well to the antibiotics. Her facial palsy and dysarthria improved rapidly. She was soon able to handle her oral secretions. On hospital Day 7, a modified barium swallow was obtained which revealed good oral control of bolus, a minimally delayed-swallow reflex, and very slight pooling in the veleculae and pyriform sinuses that was cleared with a second swallow. She was started on a pureed diet with thick liquids using a double-swallow technique.

During her acute-care hospitalization, she developed several skin tears that were treated with biocclusive dressings. She had very fragile skin. She developed some breakdown of her heels that responded well to heel protections and biocclusive dressings. Eventually, she was stabilized and transferred to the rehabilitation facility.

At that facility she remained on low-flow O_2. She was noted to have stable vital signs and was afebrile at the time of admission. She did continue to have a weak cough and poor inspiratory effort. Neurologic examination was remarkable for a subtle left central VII palsy, mild dysarthria without dysphonia, some early flexion synergy return in the left upper extremity, and left lower-extremity isolated strength which was antigravity at the hip and knee. She had trace movement of her ankle dorsi and plantar flexors. She was hyper-reflexic on the left with an upgoing toe. At admission, the nurses noted that she had had no bowel movement for five days. Admission chest x-ray revealed a resolving left lower lobe infiltrate. Admission laboratory work was remarkable for greater than 50 white blood cells and 4+ bacteria on her urinalysis. The following focus list was developed:

- Impairments in mobility, characterized by decreased ability to transfer and ambulate. Her propriperception was well preserved and at the time of admission she was minimal-to-moderate assist for transfers.

- Impairment in self-care, with decreased use of her left upper extremity. At the time of admission, however, she was already able to use it as a gross stabilizer in tasks and her sitting balance was good.

- Mild impairment with swallowing: This was rapidly improving, but because of her history of aspiration pneumonia during acute care, she was placed on aspiration precautions and followed closely by ST.

- Fragile skin: Her biocclusive dressings were all removed at the time of admission and her skin inspected.

- Constipation/urinary tract infection.

The patient, while having good strength, was initially quite fatigued and had difficulty participating in an hour and a half of PT per day. She tended to do quite well in the mornings but broke down in the afternoon. She was started on a trial of low-dose methylphenidate which greatly improved her ability to attend therapies in the afternoon. She also had a rest break scheduled after lunch which improved her fatigue level. Because of her good sitting balance and trunk strength, she rapidly obtained a contact-guard level with transfers. She was started in pregait activities and eventually was able to ambulate for household distances with a front-wheeled walker. She had difficulty with wheelchair propulsion because of a lack of an appropriately sized wheelchair secondary to her small stature. The family felt that this was not a priority because they were going to be available to help with wheelchair propulsion in the community.

The patient was able to use her left upper extremity as a gross stabilizer as she attained more isolated upper-extremity strength. She continued to have difficulty with manual dexterity but was able to incorporate her left upper extremity into self-care tasks. She was independent with self-feeding using her right hand, with grooming and hygiene, and with upper-body dressing. She required supervision for lower-body dressing secondary to decreased standing balance and supervision for functional transfers.

Her swallowing rapidly improved. Her chest remained clear. She was eventually advanced to a chopped diet with thin liquids with no further difficulties with aspiration.

The patient initially required aggressive use of laxatives and enemas to clear her impaction. Thereafter, she was started on a regular bowel program with suppository, at first daily and then every other day. She was eventually weaned off suppository and was able to defecate with just the use of a vegetable laxative and stool softener.

Her pyuria at admission had caused a low-grade fever and she was treated with antibiotics. Subsequently she developed another urinary tract infection that was again treated with a course of oral antibiotics. Her family reported that she did intermittently develop urinary tract infections prior to this hospitalization. She had a history of stress incontinence which continued to be a slight problem though no worse than previously. Once she was able to transfer more easily on and off the commode, she became continent during the day, but not overnight.

Her skin areas were all cleansed at admission and covered with opsite type dressings. She continued to develop new ones during the course of her rehabilitation, especially with transfer training. Elbow pads prevented her from banging them and helped in reducing trauma to her skin. Because of her long history of diabetes with some degree of peripheral neuropathy and fragile skin, skin surveillance was quite important. She did develop a perineal rash that was treated with topical agents and resolved. This improved greatly with the resolution in her stress incontinence.

The patient had good family support and her grandniece was designated as the caregiver and was able to complete training and act as an attendant. Because her grandniece also had to work part-time, the patient was referred to a senior day center for stroke patients in the community and spent three days a week there in their program. She had home PT and OT, initially twice weekly, to assess her mobility and self-care skills in the home and after a month was able to obtain modified independence in those areas. She continued to develop occasional urinary tract infections which were treated by her primary care physician with courses of oral antibiotics.

Case Five (JBG): Right MCA Thrombus

The patient was a 45-year-old right-handed white man, with no previous reports of hypertension, cardiac disease, hypercholesteremia, or diabetes, who had a remote history of smoking. His only medical illness in the past was a left superficial femoral vein DVT that he sustained four years previously after a 12-hour airline flight. He presented to the ER after falling out of bed. His wife noted left-sided weakness, slurred speech, and abnormal posture with his head turned to the right.

In the ER, his blood pressure was mildly elevated at 160/95 and his other vital signs were normal. Neurologic examination was significant for a left homonymous hemianopia, left-central seventh cranial nerve neuropalsy, dysarthria, and left upper-extremity greater than left lower-extremity weakness. He had significant left-side neglect and extinguished on double-simultaneous stimulation despite having relatively spared cutaneous sensation. He was very distractible and denied any problems, insisting he was fine and wanted to go home.

General laboratory work was unremarkable. EKG showed normal sinus rhythm. A CT scan of the brain was negative for hemorrhage. He was given heparin after neurologic consultation and showed some improvement in his left-sided strength during anticoagulation. His severe neglect and perceptual deficits, however, persisted. MRI/MRA performed on hospital Day 2 revealed an acute left MCA infarct with evident thrombosis of the M1 branch of the right MCA on the MRA. Carotid duplex and echocardiogram were both normal. At that point a workup for hypercoagulable state was undertaken, including rheumatoid factor, ANA, erythrocyte sedimentation rate, protein C, protein S, antithrombin III, and anticardiolipin antibody.

At the time of his admission to the rehabilitation facility he was evaluated by an interdisciplinary team. He was highly distractible, made sexually inappropriate remarks to female staff, demonstrated poor short-term memory, difficulty with carryover, and was impulsive. He continued to demonstrate dense left neglect with decreased insight into his deficits and was incontinent of bowel and bladder. His left-sided visual field cut remained quite dense, and he continued to have a moderate left hemiparesis affecting the upper extremity somewhat more than the lower extremity. On the day of his admission to the rehabilitation facility, his neurologist contacted the attending physiatrist with the information that the patient's anticardiolipin antibody had returned strongly positive. At that time a decision was made to increase his target prothrombin time and INR to a higher level and to maintain him on long-term warfarin therapy. A focus list for this patient was developed as follows:

- Behavior modification: There was a need to redirect the patient to focus more on therapeutic activities as well as to diminish his impulsivity and increase awareness of safety issues.

- Impairment in cognition, characterized by his decreased attention and concentration, impaired memory, and poor executive-functioning skills and judgment.

- Impairment in self-care and ADLs, with severe left upper-extremity paresis as well as deficits in motor-planning and visuoperceptual abilities.

- Impairment in mobility: At the time of admission, the patient was moderate assist for transfers with a tendency to push to his right side and he was nonambulatory.

Psychology, in conjunction with other team members, immediately formulated a plan for behavioral modification with consistent reinforcement to the patient by staff that his impulsive motor actions and inappropriate verbal remarks were not acceptable. He showed gradual improvement in those areas throughout hospitalization. By the end of his stay, he recognized that some of his previous behavior had been inappropriate and became somewhat remorseful, apologizing to numerous staff members. His impulsivity gradually improved, although two weeks into his hospitalization he did suffer a fall while trying to get out of bed unassisted at night; he sustained a laceration to his right ear that required a plastic surgery consultation for repair. He subsequently did have one other fall, but without injury. Secondary to some of his behavioral issues, the team felt he would definitely need ongoing 24-hour supervision.

Cognitive issues were addressed within all therapy disciplines. The patient was provided with a log book for use to compensate for memory deficits. Initially he had difficulty attending long enough to use it and his visual/perceptual dysfunctions interferred somewhat with reading and writing. Even though ST and OT worked with him on compensating for his visual field loss, these compensatory maneuvers were somewhat less than successful secondary to his visuoperceptual dysfunctions. By the end of his hospitalization, however, he was able to use his log book with fair accuracy and follow a schedule. He also was able to attend to stimuli on his left side with cues but had difficulty doing it without cues.

With respect to ADL training, again his apraxia and visuoperceptual dysfunction interferred. He was able to attain independence in grooming and hygiene using adaptive equipment and a simplified bathroom environment with less distraction. He was still minimal assist with upper- and lower-body dressing at the time of discharge secondary to difficulty incorporating hemitechnique in addition to his body-scheme distortion and motor-planning difficulties.

Initially, this patient had incontinence of both bowel and bladder. This seemed to be more on the basis of an intentional deficit on his part; and as his cognition gradually improved with a timed toileting program, he was able to achieve continence of both bowel and bladder during the day. He continued to have occasional bladder incontinence at night; this was managed with use of an external catheter, but he consistently pulled it off. Eventually, he was able to tolerate wearing the catheter at night, with decreased episodes of incontinence. He had difficulty placing a urinal during the day secondary to his apraxia but was able to become independent with its use. Functional mobility did improve to the point where he was supervised for his toilet and tub transfers with the use of adaptive equipment and his wife was trained to assist him.

The patient was initially maximal assist with transfers occasionally requiring two people secondary to his tendency to push toward his unaffected side. He showed gradual improvement in his motor function, particularly in his left lower extremity with a more moderate improvement in left upper-extremity function. He was able to use his left upper extremity as a gross assist during mobility tasks but was not able to do any fine-motor activities secondary to poor motor return in the hand. He attained a supervised status with transfers approximately two weeks into his hospitalization. Gait activities began, and at time of discharge, he was contact guard to ambulate with a quad cane and a articulated left AFO.

Despite aggressive anticoagulation and daily physical examinations, the patient developed a left common femoral vein DVT which was diagnosed on the Doppler ultrasound done secondary to acute-onset calf swelling. After consultation with his primary physician, the patient was placed at bed rest for five days with his target INR for warfarin increased to 2.5. Symptoms gradually abated; however, on his fourth day of bed rest he developed acute onset of pleuritic chest pains with mild O_2 desaturation and hypoxemia and was transferred to the acute-care facility. There a ventilation/perfusion scan showed high probability for pulmonary emboli affecting both lungs. A decision was made at that time to place a inferior venacaval filter. He returned after a five-day acute-care hospitalization and was able to resume his rehabilitation program without further incident.

Family training was ongoing with his wife during the rehabilitation hospitalization. She had significant difficulty coping with the change in their roles in the marriage. She remained in full-time employment and had to assume increased child-care responsibilities secondary to her husband's illness. Because of the ongoing need for 24-hour supervision and the lack of availability of that supervision in their home, the decision was made for the patient to be transferred to a TLC to have further rehabilitation in a more community-integrated setting prior to discharge home.

During his four-week stay, the patient did very well in transitional living and was able to move from supervised to modified-independent with all self-care and mobility. He returned home and continued to have outpatient therapy; secondary to his cognitive issues, he was unable to return to his previous job as an investment banker. Eventually, he decided to pursue further education and was able to complete a master's degree program in family therapy and is pursuing a career counseling other patients with disabilities.

Glossary

Acalculia   Loss of ability to do simple arithmetic.

Agnosia   Disorder of afferent information processing resulting in loss of ability to recognize through a particular sensory system. For example, *visual* agnosia refers to the inability to put together visual information so that it makes sense; the parts of an object may be seen but the person is unable to put it together as a "whole."

Agraphia   Inability to express thoughts in writing.

Alexia   Inability to read.

Anomia   Loss of the ability to recall the names of objects. Patients who have this disability often can speak fluently but have to use other words to describe objects. For example, a patient may say, "It's one of those things that you hold and you move it like this" (describing a hairbrush).

Anoxic encephalopathy   A lack of oxygen causing damage to the brain. This can result when blood flow is reduced or with decrease in blood oxygenation.

Apathy   A lack of interest or concern.

Aphasia   Loss of the ability to express oneself and/or to understand language. There are many different kids of *aphasia. Receptive aphasia* refers to the inability to understand what someone else is saying. This is often associated with damage to the temporal area of the brain. *Expressive aphasia* refers to an inability to express oneself. Some patients may know what they want to say but may not be able to form the words. Other patients may be able to form the words but many of the words they say may not "make sense." Expressive aphasia is often associated with the left-frontal-parietal brain lesion.

Apraxia Disorder of efferent information processing resulting in inability to perform purposeful movements even though end-organ function is preserved. Particularly refers to inability to use objects. For example, a patient may be unable to put together the proper movements to sit crosslegged on the floor or may not know what to do when handed a broom.

Aspirate Entrance of material into the airway below the level of the true vocal folds.

Astereognosia Inability to recognize things by touch.

Ataxia Inability to coordinate muscle movements. This can interfere with the person's ability to walk, talk, eat, perform self-care tasks, and work.

Attention The ability to focus on one subject or bit of information or alternate between subjects; being able to filter out the relevant from the-irrelevant information in one's environment.

Brain stem The lower portion of the brain connecting it to the spinal cord. The brain stem coordinates the body's vital functions (breathing, blood pressure, and pulse). It also houses the reticular formation, which controls consciousness, drowsiness, and attention.

Cerebellum The portion of the brain that is located below the cortex. The cerebellum is coordinates movements.

Cognition Knowing, awareness, perceiving objects, thinking, remembering ideas; the learned set of rules on which all thinking is based.

Collateral sprouting One mechanism of neural regeneration whereby new connections are formed by surviving axons.

Concentration Sustaining attention to a task over a period of time; remaining attentive.

Diplopia Seeing two images of a single object ("double vision").

Disability Any restriction or lack of an ability to perform an activity in the manner or within the range considered normal for a human being.

Disinhibition The inability to control or inhibit impulses and emotions.

Dysarthria   Difficulty forming or articulating words. This may be caused by damage to the motor areas of the cortex or damage to the brain stem. Dysarthric speech is slurred and poorly enunciated.

Dysphagia   Swallowing dysfunction.

Emotional lability (emotionalism)   Exhibiting rapid and drastic changes in emotions; quickly becoming angry, sad, silly, or happy, and being extreme in showing these emotions.

Flaccidity   Muscles that feel soft and lax.

Handicap   A disadvantage for a given individual, resulting from an impairment or a disability that limits or prevents the fulfillment of a role that is normal (depending on age, sex, and social and cultural factors) for that individual.

Hemiparesis   Weakness of one side of the body (or part of it) because of an injury to the motor areas of the brain.

Hemiplegia   Complete paralysis of one side.

Homonymous hemianopsia   Loss of vision in corresponding halves of the visual fields, due to interruption of the visual pathway behind the optic chiasm.

Hypertonia   Increased tone, manifested as increased resistance to passive muscle stretch; stiffness.

Hypotonia   Decreased tone, manifested as decreased resistance to passive muscle stretch; floppiness.

Impairment   Any loss or abnormality of psychological, physical, or anatomical structure or function.

Inflexibility   The inability to adjust to everyday changes in routines, usually related to injury to the frontal lobes. Some head-injured persons may have little difficulty following a structured routine but may exhibit sudden frustration and confusion when their routine is changed.

Judgment   The process of forming an opinion, based on an evaluation of the situation at hand. "Good" judgment refers to choosing the optimal available course. Judgment involves cognitive skills, personal values and preferences, and insights into an individual's abilities and disabilities. For example, a patient with judgment deficits may be able to make decisions, but the decisions may be unsafe or unsuccessful.

Kinesiology   Study of movement.

Memory   The process of perceiving information, organizing and storing it, and retrieving it at a later time as needed. Memory is a complex function that involves many parts of the brain working together There are different "types" of memory, including *immediate* (repeating a phone number), *recent* (recalling what occurred the previous day) and *remote* (recalling the name of a childhood friend).

Mobile arm support   Upper-extremity orthosis that translates proximal strength to distal muscles, thereby facilitating forearm movement for tasks such as feeding; often attaches to chair.

Neural unmasking   One method of neural recovery whereby "dominant" neural pathways are activated and/or used in new ways.

Neuromuscular facilitation   Any exercise or positioning method that results in muscle contraction or improved posture because of application of external stimuli such as vibration or touch; often used specifically in regard to proprioceptive neuromuscular facilitation (PNF).

Odynophagia   Partial swallowing.

Perseveration   Becoming "stuck" on one word or task and not being able to switch back and forth or go on to the next word/task. (For example, a patient may be asked to draw a circle on a piece of paper. He may then be asked to draw a square, but instead continues drawing circles.)

Ptosis   Eyelid droop.

Problem solving   The ability to evaluate all of the factors involved when faced with a problem, and to generate and evaluate possible solutions. Patients with deficits in this area may "freeze" when faced with a problem; that is, they may not be able to think of possible solutions and instead respond by doing nothing.

Quadrantanopsias   Vision deficit involving one or more quadrants of the visual field.

Reflex sympathetic dystrophy   Syndrome of sympathetic activation causing pain, swelling, vasomotor changes, and loss of function in injured body part. After stroke, upper extremity reflex sympathetic dystrophy is often called *shoulder–hand syndrome.*

Spasticity   Upper-motor neuron syndrome complex including increase in muscle tone, resistance to passive muscle stretch, and hyperreflexia. A patient with spasticity may look "curled up," with her or his arms held close to the chest, or she or he may appear very stiff.

Spontaneous recovery   The recovery that takes place spontaneously as the brain heals; this type of recovery occurs early in the recovery process, with or without rehabilitation. It is often difficult to know how much improvement is spontaneous and how much is due to rehabilitative interventions.

Unilateral neglect   Not responding to things on one side. This usually occurs on the side opposite from the location of injury (right-sided brain injury, neglect left side). Some patients only exhibit this when both sides of the body are being touched at once. In extreme cases, the patient may not bathe, dress, or acknowledge one side of his body.

Visual-field deficit   Disorder of visual information processing because of lesion(s) in the retina to the occipital lobes.

Note: Some of the definitions here are from The Family Guide to the Rehabilitation of the Severely Brain-Injured Patient, 1989, which is under copyright protection. Reprinted with permission from Healthcare Rehabilitation Center, Austin, TX. The definitions are not highly technical to facilitate understanding.

Index

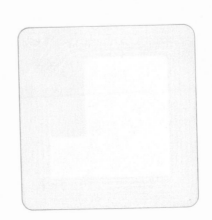